The Decline of American Medicine

3/9/96

Dear Jack & Pat:

Thank you for your interest in this little book. Wouldn't it be great if the health care system were to get better?

Michael Rosenblum

The Decline of American Medicine

✦

Where Have All the Doctors Gone?

Michael Rosenblum M.D.

iUniverse, Inc.
New York Lincoln Shanghai

The Decline of American Medicine
Where Have All the Doctors Gone?

iUniverse, Inc.

For information address:
iUniverse, Inc.
2021 Pine Lake Road, Suite 100
Lincoln, NE 68512
www.iuniverse.com

ISBN: 0-595-28419-1

Printed in the United States of America

Contents

Acknowledgements

My wife Elaine, always supportive of my projects, provided a profusion of assistance and ideas.

My former office manager, Sheila Ulmer, was the first to point out to me, ten years before I began this manuscript, that the government and insurance companies "do not want you to practice medicine."

Helen Doughty, medical librarian, provided valuable research assistance.

The late Peter Shaw inspired me to write, and made an effort to make it readable.

The author would also like to thank the following for their contributions and their willingness to be interviewed: Joyce Abrams RN, Kristine Anderson RN, Dan Barry, Mel Belsky M.D., Mark Christiansen M.D., Al Ewing, Andrew Kives M.D., Bernard Larner M.D., Ken Meehan, Jay Nathan, Pamela Packard RN, Barbara Paul M.D., Annie Raskin, Ron Relic, Lee Robbins PhD, Gerald N. Rogan M.D., Craig Sadur M.D., Gina Sarbo RN, Robert W. Sosna, Richard Dean Smith M.D., George Spradling, Penelope A.Wells DrPH, Charles Wohl M.D.. Equal thanks go to those who have chosen to remain anonymous.

Prologue: 1969

"So, you're going to medical school and you're going to study to be a doctor."
    "Yeah."
    "Well, you're gonna have to work very hard, but once you finish your studies, you'll never have to worry about money."

In The Trenches: 1973

"Code Blue[1], Emergency Room…" I had picked up the phone in the on-call room while still asleep, and now I started to remember that I had to MOVE. The clock next to the bed said 1:59. After 40 hours of non-stop patient care, the resident, Charlie, had given his intern a break. I had been permitted to collapse into a dreamless coma in the on-call room, still dressed, at midnight, but the magic two-hour break was over. I ran in my stale white intern pants and smock to the ER, still fighting off the remnants of a deep and exhausted sleep. An older male patient was in cardiac arrest, and Charlie was running the Code, that is, directing the procedures designed to restart heartbeat and breathing, as residents do while on call. So, in the wee hours of a humid July Monday in Massachusetts in 1973 I dutifully responded to the command "Pump!" from Charlie and performed external chest compression. Meanwhile, he inserted a tube in the patient's windpipe and attempted to ventilate the patient with a big black balloon called an Ambu-Bag, which he squeezed rhythmically in an effort to force air into the patient's lungs. It was a futile effort. After 45 minutes of external chest compression and mechanical breathing, three jolts of electric shock to the heart, an injection of epinephrine directly into the heart, and a large dose of sweat, we pronounced the patient dead, Charlie went to talk to the family to try to get permission for an autopsy, and I went on to the next critical problem.

It was a weekend to remember. I have never had one quite as difficult since then. For 48 hours, minus the two-hour sleep, I was on the run. There were 23 seriously ill patients to admit to the hospital. There were approximately 30 Code Blue situations. At night, I had to start and restart all the IV's for perhaps 100 patients in the 360-bed hospital. Constant calls about unstable patients kept me busy minute to minute. Meals were quickly inhaled in the hospital cafeteria, with caloric supplementation from whatever junk food was lying around the back of the nurses' stations on each floor. My reward for making it to Monday 8 AM was not rest, but a day's work on my regular weekday ward, making rounds on

---

1. "Code Blue" is the emergency call to designated members of the hospital staff to respond to a patient in cardiac arrest.

patients, and admitting several more to the hospital with a detailed history and physical exam. While attending a couple of hour-long conferences, I nodded off in my seat. I finally shuffled out of the hospital into the humid evening air, shell-shocked and physically exhausted after 60 hours in the building. My wife was quite understanding of my state, and didn't complain when I was asleep by 8 PM, dreaming of insoluble medical crises.

I was paid about $10,000 per year for this training in medicine, working 100 hours per week, and missing approximately one night of sleep in three. The weeknight on call nights came one at a time, so the workday was only 36 hours, as opposed to every third weekend with its 48 hour stretch on call with a busy Monday attached. Sometimes, the hospital was relatively quiet and I had two or three hours of uninterrupted sleep in the on-call room for a night.

My elders in the profession brushed off any complaints by pointing out that they had to be on-call every other night when they were interns, and that I had it easy with one night in three. "The only problem with being on-call every other night is that you miss half of the good cases." One doctor who did his internship in India pointed out that he was indeed "interned" for the whole year, not leaving the hospital premises and being on call continuously. I was told, "Well, you get a little tired, but think of all the people you are helping," and, "This is what it is like to be a doctor."

My contact with the world of the non-hospitalized patients was very limited initially. I went to a neighborhood clinic one afternoon or one evening per week. There were minor problems to diagnose and treat, interspersed with the occasional ambulatory but seriously ill patient who needed to be sent to the hospital. I was probably viewed as a brusque and arrogant young doctor by the patients. Outpatient clinic was something to be taken care of as rapidly as possible. The patients were not part of a long-term practice with long-term relationships with the doctor. Only in retrospect can I see what was lacking in the care I provided. The important goal then was to return to the hospital and learn the new technology for caring for the critically ill.

"Everyone Gets Everything"

"Health care, a right not a privilege" was the presumption in medical training in the late 1960s and early 1970s. A clinical work-up of a patient's symptoms therefore left no stone unturned and no test undone. As residents-in-training, a favorite ploy of our teachers was to find a test we had not thought of doing in the search for uncommon causes of a common disease. Someone else would pay for the patient's care, and that was not our concern as his or her doctor. Medical professors never mentioned the economics of health care. Such discussion was considered inappropriate and politically incorrect.

I look back on those days with wonder that some of our patients survived the testing we did to them. If there was fluid on a joint or fluid in a body cavity, that fluid had to be reached with a big needle and drained so that a sample of it could be sent to the laboratory for testing. If there was a pain, then the region of the body with the pain was studied with an X-ray. Hospitalized patients were rendered anemic due to the constant daily withdrawal of blood samples for testing. Thorough and complete study of every abnormality of every patient was what we doctors-in-training were to strive for. Terms like "efficiency" were not part of the daily vocabulary. Patients spent days or weeks lying around the hospital waiting for "tests." Some private insurers noted hospital stays of many weeks for patients who were not seriously ill. There were early attempts at "utilization review" by a few private health insurance companies. I remember several elderly, semi-retired M.D.s who were paid by the insurance companies to look at the charts of hospital inpatients and determine whether there was "medical necessity" for continued hospitalization. On occasion, an insurance company used the data gathered to tell the patient and primary doctor that the hospitalization would not be covered beyond a certain date. However, hospital stays tended to be long, and many patients in the hospital were able to walk and eat under their own power. The idea of being hospitalized for a "rest" and for "tests" was a perfectly acceptable use of a hospitalization to the general public, and the insurance companies only protested the most flagrantly unnecessary stays in the facility.

I am reminded of an experience I had in 1971. I was doing a medical student clinical clerkship on the gynecology service of a university hospital. Medical students tagged along with the residents, feeling clumsy and inept, trying to learn the many diseases in each specialty area and their treatments. Some of the hours of each day were spent doing "scut work," such as minding tubes, running tests, and writing chart notes. An unfortunate woman in her 40s required irrigation of her abdomen three times a day. She had ovarian cancer, with little hope of recovery. The malignant cells were slowly growing through the abdominal cavity, following surgery to remove as much of the cancer as possible. Perhaps in part due to the debilitating effects of chemotherapy, the surgical wound had broken down, creating artificial openings between the peritoneal cavity in the abdomen and the outside. Infection was festering in the abdomen, and several times each day a soupy mixture of pus and half-dead tumor tissue had to be irrigated from the abdomen, a sort of hosing out of the debris with a large syringe and a stream of lukewarm saline solution. This task was delegated to me.

I remember writing a note in the patient's chart at the nurses' station, something like "peritoneal cavity irrigated with 300 ml normal saline" and signing my name and MS III (indicating I was a third-year medical student). There were other medical students and several residents around the nurses' station, writing in the charts. The chart of the patient with the ovarian cancer had a sticker on its metal cover, "chart thinned," with 14 separate dates noted in pencil on the sticker. I realized that the patient had been on this hospital floor for more than eight months, slowly getting worse, now with draining holes in her belly. I mumbled an offhand conclusion to the resident, standing next to me, leaning on the counter: "This patient has been here for more than eight months, and her hospital bill must be huge."

The resident, a serious crew-cut type in a scrub suit, gasped and lashed out angrily in a loud voice, "We *never* talk about money when we are dealing with someone's hospital care! Health is more precious than any amount of money. Besides, insurance takes care of *everything.*"

And that is how I learned that unlimited funding for all the necessary and almost necessary tests and surgeries was available, paid for by mysterious and benevolent insurance companies. I only had to worry about caring for the patient. Someone else would deal with the cost.

Years have passed and I am astounded at how the cycle has gone to the opposite extreme. For those who are not in the health professions, it is difficult to realize how far we have gone as a society in worrying about the finances first and the patient last. I will try to explain some of the landmark events that have led to a dehumanized and deprofessionalized health care system.

The Goose with the Golden Eggs

Title XVIII of the Social Security Act, commonly known as "Medicare," was passed in 1965. It was a feature of President Lyndon B. Johnson's "Great Society" and established a health insurance program for persons over 65. When implemented in 1966, there were more than 19 million persons enrolled in the program. It consisted of Part A, Hospital Insurance, automatically provided to persons 65 and over, and financed through a payroll tax paid by workers and their employers. Part B, Supplementary Medical Insurance, was optional, with a monthly premium, and was to cover services outside the hospital. The premiums, deducted from a person's Social Security check, covered about half of the cost of Part B, with the remainder coming from general tax revenues.

Within several years of its inception, the budget for Medicare services was far exceeding expectations. The trust fund established to fund Part A was rapidly depleted, and payroll tax rates to finance Social Security and Medicare climbed steadily.

Looking back on that early era of Medicare, one can say that the profession was blessed with a goose laying golden eggs. A service performed in a hospital for a patient over 65 years of age was well reimbursed, no questions asked. Or at least, only relatively simple paperwork was required compared to that required later. The vast majority of hardworking doctors billed honestly for their services. Outright fraud, that is, billing for services never rendered or surgery not actually done was rare. But the vast flow of federal money was helping to finance new modern hospitals, and major medical teaching programs, and providing an opportunity for high-tech, expensive procedures to proliferate rapidly. The sicker, older population needed these services more than younger patients. I guess it is true that the older one gets, the more that things break, even in health-conscious people who try to take good care of themselves.

I am reminded of the day during my residency when several of my white-coated colleagues and I were gathered outside the endoscopy room at our hospital. Endoscopy is the use of flexible, fiberoptic instruments to look inside the stomach and intestines. A specialist called a gastroenterologist performs the procedure. Technically, a gastroenterologist (the "GI" man) is a "subspecialist" in one organ system of the body, the digestive tract. To become a gastroenterologist requires five years of training after medical school, including three years of residency in Internal Medicine, and two years of a postdoctoral fellowship in gastroenterology.

The gastroenterologist emerged from the procedure room to discuss a puzzling case with the residents. "The upper GI endoscopy is normal," he told us. He had inserted a scope in the sedated, elderly patient through the mouth and down into the stomach and had not found an ulcer or cancer, conditions we suspected might be causing the patient's anemia. "By the way, gentlemen, what is the indication for [reason for performing] an upper GI endoscopy?" He was quizzing us, so we began to list the conditions that the endoscopy would help to diagnose. "No, no!" he interrupted us, "The indication for an upper GI endoscopy is the presence of a stomach." In other words, any patient with any vague symptom would get the procedure. This was meant as a joke, the kind of sarcastic gallows humor that is common in the hospital setting, hopefully out of earshot of the patient. But the sarcastic comment had an element of truth. That is, Medicare and other insurers readily paid for this expensive new diagnostic procedure. One merely had to fill in the diagnosis "abdominal pain" on the form to be sent to the insurer, and the insurance company would make a substantial payment for doing the procedure.

There are many stomachs out there across the land, and a hurting tummy happens to most of us now and then. So, one can readily do the arithmetic and realize that if each and every citizen had an upper GI endoscopy each year, we could consume most of the health care budget in the United States with this one high-tech procedure. Obviously, not every stomach gets scoped, but it is true that the older a patient is, the more likely he is to need the procedure. So among the population of Medicare age, many upper GI endoscopies are performed. In the Golden Era of Medicare, in the late 1960s and 1970s, the number of procedures like these steadily rose. Some of the endoscopies were true emergencies, such as in a case of bleeding from the stomach or in a patient with intractable pain and weight loss. Many of the patients were done in less urgent situations. A patient with a bellyache of several weeks duration might have a harmless stomach irritation from "stress," or might have a more serious problem like an ulcer or a tumor. In the Golden Era, the expensive new test that could rapidly diagnose the small fraction of patients with a serious problem was performed readily if even minor symptoms were present. Lavish use of the new scope technology prompted the cynical comment from my mentor that the procedure is performed if there is the presence of a stomach.

Collectively, the unexpectedly great volume of medical services under Medicare reimbursement had a negative effect: We doctors wrung the neck of the goose laying the golden eggs, and killed it. In the late 1960s, it would have been impossible to foresee that such a bounty of health care funding could lead to dire results. The full consequences of our actions are still being played out, as I will delineate later. However, in the Golden Age of Medicare, from approximately 1965 to 1983, doctors became accustomed to the elderly being provided with all necessary medical services, and the elderly became accustomed to the entitlement. In fact, some patients would become irate when informed that there were deductibles or co-payments required for a particular medical service. "Why doesn't Medicare pay for this?"

Economists have pointed out with the often-quoted cliché that "There is no such thing as a free lunch." A corollary might be, "All good entitlements must end some day." Medicare in principle was a great idea. Many impoverished retired folks, living from month to month on a Social Security check or small pension, could not afford medical care until they were desperately ill. Then, when it was impossible to care for them at home, their family trundled them off to a county hospital. Ultimately, they had to be placed in a county nursing facility where they remained until they died.

Once an entitlement is established, and people become accustomed to the benefits it provides, it is very difficult to reduce or remove the services provided for "free." It is human nature to become used to the free lunch, paid for by someone else, and to feel "ripped off" when it is no longer provided. Teenagers provided with expensive automobiles by their suburban parents begin to think that having a car, paid for by someone else, filled with gasoline using a parent's credit card, is a standard benefit for commuting to high school. By detaching the valuable product or service from any sense of its value in money or hours of labor, we actually demean the sense of self-worth of the person receiving it. So it became with Medicare, as technology advanced through the 1960s and 1970s, and the trust fund was drained. Patients expected the best of care, and the cost was not a concern to them.

On the other hand, some political figures and health policy makers have advocated a health care system for the entire U.S. population paid for by a trust fund like Medicare. Money from private insurance plans would be pooled into the trust fund under this type of "single-payer" system. During the Clinton presidency, a strong effort in Congress to introduce such a plan was blown away by a consortium of insurance company and health management company interests. To provide even a simple package of basic health services to all citizens through a single-payer plan would drastically increase overall health care expenditures in the United States. Notwithstanding this economic reality, politicians promoting single-payer plans often exhort the public to support "good health care for all at a lower overall cost than we now pay with our hodgepodge of insurance plans." There is an appeal to our sense of egalitarianism. We can provide something essential and potentially life-saving to those who lack it. The problem is, we have already tried this out for seniors, since the inception of Medicare in 1965. The trust fund backing Medicare Part A benefits has been depleted, despite huge increases in Social Security taxes to pay for the funding of it. The budgetary drain of the general tax revenues required to fund Part B has become an economic and political issue of significant proportions. We need to fix the existing system before we extend it to the entire population. Otherwise, we face ever-tighter cost controls, ever more convoluted federal regulations, and scarcity of the essential services we supposedly are paying for through our rising taxes. But let me describe some of the cost containment measures already in place, now that the Golden Goose is dead.

The PPO

The rise in health insurance premiums became a national issue by the early 1980s. In the early era of employer-based health insurance, monthly or quarterly premiums were a comparatively cheap benefit for employees. While there was a steady rise in health insurance premium costs in the 1950s and through the early 1960s, a more vigorous acceleration occurred in the later 1960s. Many factors contributed to this rise. The new Medicare and Medicaid programs, crafted under the liberal democratic policies of the Lyndon B. Johnson presidency, began to pour billions of dollars into the health care system. New medical schools and residency training programs were subsidized. Hospital construction was subsidized. The United States began to approach the ideal of health care access for all, paid for by either a government or a private insurance policy. In medical school, we heard the credo of the times: "Health care is a right, not a privilege." This phrase grates against my brain like chalk on an old-fashioned blackboard. Other quotes from that era around 1970 that still float through my head include, "This is medicine…every patient gets everything and we never concern ourselves with the cost," and, "Don't worry! Insurance will pay for it." It was a time of *carte blanche* coverage of the costs by a benevolent third-party. There was a patina of goodness and entitlement on the whole process, compared to what ensued in subsequent years.

Major changes began that marked an end to the easy times of the "nifty" 50s and 60s in the U.S. economy in 1970. The centerpiece of our economy, old industrial giants making steel and automobiles, began to lose market share to more competitive foreign manufacturers, operating out of new efficient plants with cheaper labor. Inflation accelerated, as the infusion of the federal dollars of the Johnson Great Society era of "guns and butter," that is, the Vietnam War and vast new social programs, moved through the economy. New medical specialties and subspecialties, and emerging new medical technologies, raised the per capita health care cost tremendously. Medical care is labor intensive, and the sicker you are, the more you need high-paid nurses, technicians, and doctors. As medical costs zoomed nationally, and the still-new Medicare program accelerated in expenditures at a rate far in excess of projections, economists began to take notice. We were still in the era of fee-for-service medicine for the vast majority of patients. There was complete choice of doctors and hospitals, and a significant proportion of care took place in the doctor's office, with predominance of solo doctors and small groups of doctors.

In 1973 and 1974, economic shock waves rocked the nation. An embargo on Mideast oil exports caused the sudden rampant inflation of fuel costs and made for a very cold winter in the U.S. Midwest and Northeast. Manufacturing facilities shut down, unable to pay for rising fuel costs. Unemployment soared, and state unemployment checks did not pay for the increased costs of home heating. I was living in Massachusetts at the time, and enjoyed social events in friends' homes with the interior temperature at 45 degrees Fahrenheit. At the hospital, we treated cases of carbon monoxide poisoning as people tried to stay warm burning charcoal indoors or wrapping their houses in layers of heavy plastic. The Nixon administration imposed a wage and price freeze, but this failed to control inflation as black market trading of goods and services became rampant. Gasoline prices soared from around 30 cents per gallon to more than a dollar per gallon, with shortages leading to long lines at gas stations, and a limited allocation, such as 4 or 8 gallons, once you reached the pump.

Former manufacturing centers, like Pittsburgh and Cleveland, became the "rust belt" of the United States. A generation of assembly line and plant workers, accustomed to a union wage scale and lifetime employment with full benefits, suddenly found itself living on unemployment checks. Many waited in vain for the mills to reopen, but it was nearly a generation before rehabilitation of the plants began, often with a conversion to high-tech automated facilities or to office and shopping space. In the interim, the prolonged recession of the 1970s and early 1980s swelled the ranks of those receiving health care under federally funded Medicaid programs and helped drive the budget for federal programs to unexpected heights in an era of declining tax revenue.

The rhetoric from Washington in the early 1980s began to have a new message. "The rising cost of health care is making the United States less competitive in the world marketplace." The cost of worker health insurance premiums in the United States was quoted as many hundreds of dollars per new automobile. The percentage of the gross domestic product, the value of all goods and services produced in the nation, devoted to health care had crossed the 10 percent mark and was rising rapidly. Liberal academic types pointed to socialist democracies in Western Europe that provided health care for all citizens using 6 or 8 percent of the gross domestic product. Doctors, hospitals, and university medical centers were accused of being wasteful and inefficient in the United States, and the rising number of uninsured and underinsured persons was widely publicized as a shameful national crisis.

And so a coalition of experts including economists, insurance executives and representatives of government agencies developed a new catch phrase to present a proposed solution: "Managed Care." In reality, it was "Managed Cost," but the concept of improved efficient care at a savings was "embraced" by mesmerized leaders of academic medicine as a way out of the "crisis" in health care cost and availability.

The first type of cost-reduction effort to sweep the nation was the preferred provider organization, or PPO. This was the first major change in health insurance since the straight indemnity type of insurance, like the traditional Blue Cross and Blue Shield plans, which became widespread starting in the 1950s, and the original Medicare program as passed in 1965.

In the PPO version of health insurance, the patient receives a list of "preferred" hospitals and doctors. A small co-payment by the patient is required to see the doctor, after annual deductibles are met. The doctor has signed a contract with the PPO to provide services at a discount to "market" rates, as has the hospital. Defining a free-market rate for health care services has become a very fuzzy process over the last two decades, but the initial discount in the 1980s was 15 to 30 percent from usual fees.

In California, the entry of the PPOs in the early 1980s was gradual. The new technology boom in the Silicon Valley was getting underway. Initially, much of the manufacturing of chip and computer components was being done in the area, so there was a non-union, semi-skilled labor force of assemblers working there. Employers scrambled to find the cheapest possible health insurance plans for their employees as health insurance premiums continued to escalate. PPOs were the answer.

Companies offering medical insurance saw a new opportunity to compete for market share with a greater profit margin. Dollars drove the system, and there were dollars to be made corralling health care "providers" into the new way of doing business. I doubt that there were any altruistic concerns in the boardrooms of leading insurance companies. Here was the new and unexploited market for cheaper health care coverage with better margins. "Let's go for it" was the plan. The new plans were pitched at medical staff meetings at hospitals. The talented people recruited to tout the benefits to physicians and hospitals impressed me with their expertise in high-powered soft sell. I went to the meetings, which were well attended by the doctors. The pitchmen had slides with charts and graphs, perfect haircuts, $800 suits, and a skillfully delivered message: "Sign on, and you won't have to worry about losing patients. Don't worry! You may have to see a few more patients each week to make up for the discount in fees, but sign on and we'll take care of you."

Doctors and hospitals did gradually sign on, hoping to "maintain patient base and make up the discount on volume." Personally, I tried to avoid signing these contracts to give away my services at a discount, but many of my colleagues shrugged their shoulders and said, "I have no choice." I joked sarcastically that PPO actually stands for "Professional Pimping Organization." I received laughs as I told my fellow M.D.s, "The pimps get the first 30 percent, and you're getting beat up in the street." They signed anyway, fearing the loss of patients if they did not. Gradual erosion of physician income began in those years, as fee increases no longer kept up with rising practice expenses and inflation. Greed within the profession, manifested as pumping the maximum fees out of the old-style indemnity health insurance plans, was now replaced by fear, the fear of losing patients and of losing income. In an ideal world, behavior would not be driven by the greed-to-fear ratio. In the real world of business, greed and fear are the controlling forces of behavior. Greed could be found in the newly emerging health management companies, bent on improving the bottom line by controlling the dollars that formerly went to patient care. To a doctor, the fear of losing a significant fraction of one's patients led to the signing of contracts to provide care at a discount. Self-respect declined, and, along with it, the caring attitude of the professional waned. There was a loss of being in control of one's professional work. But more profound losses would come later.

HMOs and Capitation

The invasion of Kuwait by Iraq in 1990 was associated with a brief but intense business recession in the United States. Health care costs continued to escalate, and the feared threshold of health care consuming more than 10 percent of the gross domestic product had been crossed. And so, the medical marketplace was ripe for the next phase of the managed care revolution, "capitation." The men in expensive suits from the insurance companies were out and about once again, talking to hospital administrators and groups of doctors about the new form of insurance, the HMO or "health maintenance organization." The original HMO in California, Kaiser Health Plan, had been around for 45 years, but it was "closed panel." Patient members could only be seen in Kaiser Hospitals and by Kaiser doctors. The new HMO structures were open; that is, there was a choice of hospitals and their affiliated doctors from whom the patient could receive covered services. The middlemen in these operations were initially existing health insurance companies, but many of these evolved into health management corporations. They no longer indemnified patients; that is, they no longer accepted the risk of the cost of illness. Rather, they collected premiums from patients or their employers and doled out some of this money as capitation pools for doctor and hospital services. In effect, a preset amount per month, or "capitation rate," was provided in separate pools to hospitals for hospital charges and to doctor groups for physician charges. Physicians were encouraged to merge into ever-larger groups to expand their market share and receive larger volumes of capitation payments for "covered lives." Patients were no longer real people. Now they were an accounting entity with a monthly value to the doctor. For the primary care internist or family practitioner, the monthly fee was typically $11 per month per covered life. However, $3 of this fee was withheld by the management company as an incentive to "decrease utilization" of patient services. The physician would receive an incentive check for using less than some benchmark quantity of patient visits, lab tests, and X-ray studies. Expensive procedures would require "preauthorization," in which the doctor or his staff would call an 800 number, wait on hold, and talk to a clerk who would permit or decline the advanced permission needed for coverage of the procedure. I wonder how many millions of hours of time have been wasted with pre-authorization phone calls. The hassle of getting pre-authorization for proposed procedures certainly discourages utilization, which is the desired effect. With statistics showing an initial reduction in utilization of services, the plan can market itself as providing "efficient, cost-effective health care." Initially, the management companies running the HMO schemes touted their efficiency and ignored the delayed treatment, minimized treatment, or no treatment patients received under their plans. Bewildered patients, when finally sick enough, headed to the emergency rooms. The payment for services was denied by the plan, on grounds that care could have been received in a doctor's office. Many state legislatures sprang into action, passing legislation mandating coverage of emergencies as defined by "any prudent lay person."

This HMO scenario was very confusing to those not in the health field, and somewhat obscure even to those who signed the contracts. To me, the key point was that doctors were no longer rewarded for seeing sick people and taking care of them. Now there were strong financial incentives to not treat or to undertreat the patient. A whole new language of buzzwords filled the marketing brochures, and even distinguished academic medical journals had special articles on the wonders of capitation. It was described as a "miraculous" method of reigning in out-of-control health care spending.

One geographic area that experienced an almost overnight switch from indemnity insurance to HMO insurance was Madison, Wisconsin. Being the capital of the state and home of a large state university, the majority of employees and their families were state employees. Their choices of health insurance were changed to HMOs. Local doctors and hospitals had no choice but to sign up for the capitated HMO plans, or risk seeing most of their patients migrate to other facilities. The effect on doctor income was immediate and profound. Running a solo doctor office or a small group office typically involved overhead of around 50 percent. A sudden cut in income of 20 percent would produce a drop in net income of 40 percent, a noticeable decline for the doctor and his family. The rules under the capitated plans were very difficult for doctors. The monthly capitated rate, or fixed-fee payment per patient, included a "withhold," a 30 percent pool of money held back which was promised as a year-end bonus if certain consultations and tests were performed fewer times than some benchmark level defined by the insurance company. This was a direct conflict of interest for the doctor, who had to choose between being thorough and professional in his or her care of the patient and reducing the level of services provided to assure economic survival. In the Madison, Wisconsin area, some doctor groups were told in the early years of capitation that they had utilized such an excessive amount of services that they would not get the "withhold" at the end of the year. Also, under the terms of the contract, they actually owed money to the insurance companies for ordering too many consultations. The insurance companies providing health plans to residents of the area gradually combined into a few large entities, so a doctor group refusing to sign a bad contract lost a significant proportion of its patients.

In discussing the pros and cons of capitated care and HMO plans, I find it useful to consider the difference between profit motive and greed. Financial remuneration is a powerful motivator. Is it unethical to be compensated for one's training and experience? Should we expect doctors to perform difficult procedures, which require years of training to learn to do well, for little or no reward? To the extent that market forces operated during the peak years of the solo general practitioner, there was reward for hard work, and doctors were considered distinguished professionals, worthy of a relatively high income. The new equation in delivering health care was the ratio of greed to fear.

Consider the situation that developed with the arrival of the HMOs. There was big money in setting up these plans, but not for doctors. The big bucks were up for grabs to competing health management companies, the new breed of "insurance" company that no longer assumed any risk for the costs of health care. The power moved to the management companies that could rustle up the largest numbers of "capitated lives." The cost of premiums paid by the employer was initially well below the rates for an indemnity or a PPO type of health insurance. The savings resulted from supplying the doctors and hospitals with too little money to adequately care for the patients in the HMO: The management companies took a significant proportion of the money spent by employers and patients for the plans off the top. However, they were most successful in signing on doctors and hospitals to the plans, by exploiting the fear of losing large numbers of patients to other providers of care. Initially, doctors and hospitals fantasized that a new effort at improving operating efficiency would reduce their overhead and allow profitability despite the low payments per patient per month.

Now, the great motivator of money was detached from the goal of providing good care to patients. For the management companies, their initial success in promoting HMOs depended upon getting a large pool of "capitated lives" by offering very low premiums compared to the other types of health insurance plans. For the doctor groups, staying alive financially no longer depended upon being accessible to patients and providing good care in a timely fashion. Rather, the money provided per patient per month needed to be conserved by reducing the amount of care. Tests were minimized and postponed. Phone receptionists at doctors' offices were replaced by voice mail systems. The front lines of health care became decidedly less friendly while the doctors were trying to conserve the dollars received from the capitation pools. The dollars withheld from "greedy" doctors were not used in patient care, but ultimately went to the shareholders of the publicly-traded health management companies. The largest individual shareholders were in many cases the officers and members of the Boards of Directors of these companies. In the heady days of the 1990s stock market boom, a number of executives saw the value of their shares rise to the hundreds of millions of dollars.

In California, I did not sign any HMO contracts to receive monthly capitation payments for patient care. I found myself unable to give up the attitude that the patient comes first. A sick person needs care quickly, often at high expense. In effect, a doctor gives up his professional identity when operating under capitation. He is now working to benefit a new set of customers, the employer and the health management company of the employer. The fewer services he provides to each "capitated life," the more income he retains from the capitation fees. The management company can gin up statistics on "efficient care at lower cost" and market the program to additional employers. Doctors who tried to shore up their sagging incomes in the early 1990s in California had to scramble to develop a whole new practice culture. I personally observed some disgusting and unprofessional behavior around me. Good doctors, who used to welcome paying patients to their offices, now had a population of "capitated lives" comprising perhaps half of their patients. The staff member answering the office phone now had the new task of ascertaining a patient's health plan type when they called for an appointment. If the patient had a traditional fee-for–service indemnity coverage or PPO coverage, they were seen as soon as possible for an urgent complaint. If the patient had HMO coverage, an effort was made to service their problem by phone or temporize on the appointment. Another option, which I will discuss further, was to tell the patient to go the emergency room. The emergency room M.D.s operated under a separate capitation pool, and therefore would see the patient without any negative financial impact on the primary physician.

The negative effects of capitation continue to work their way through the medical profession. In the last few years of my practice career, I saw professionalism replaced by battles for a dwindling supply of dollars for health care. The insurers basically told the doctors and the hospital, "Here's a supply of bucks, representing such-and-such a sum per capitated life per month. Now, you decide how to utilize this money wisely and provide the needed care cheaply and efficiently. And, oh yes, we will ask you to monitor the 'clinical outcomes' for quality control, using some of this money we are giving you, in order to measure whether you are providing adequate care."

Well, the money allocated is not adequate for good care, and I have seen once proud and independent professionals reduced to the status of junkyard dogs, fighting for scraps thrown over the fence. It is an ugly scene, but when pressed to explain their participation in capitated plans, a doctor will shrug his or her shoulders and say something like, "I have no choice. I have a family and a mortgage and college tuition to worry about."

One of the enabling factors for the survival of HMOs is contained in Federal laws collectively known as the Employee Retirement Security Act of 1974 (ERISA). Among its many provisions that supposedly protect employee benefits are a set of rules exempting employers, insurers, HMOs, and third-party health benefit plan administrators from state law personal injury and wrongful death lawsuits. Notice that doctors are not on the list of those exempted. Basically, ERISA sets up the rules as follows: It allows employers to save tremendous benefit dollars by herding their employees into a choice of HMO plans. The employees are now "capitated lives" in a health plan, rather than insured patients. The health plan management company can pay out a drastically reduced per life per month fixed fee to a designated doctor and hospital, who then assume all risk, fiscal and professional, for the care of the capitated lives. No wonder the average working person can no longer easily get quality health care! The doctor is paid *not* to see the patient. If the patient is sick enough to require hospitalization, each day there costs the hospital money. The fixed fee per member per month has already been paid. The cartoon image of the sick patient being discharged on a stretcher, still in a hospital gown, with an IV still attached is amazingly close to reality. Of course, this assumes that the patient has survived their hospital stay. The "dumbing down" of hospital staff to reduce labor costs has led to increased errors in care. One study showed a 7 percent increase in the chance of a patient dying for each additional patient added to a nurse's work load.[1] These data have generated sufficient anguish in the lay press[2] that we now have new federal legislation creating a new agency and new paperwork to track errors in hospital care. The obvious solution of providing adequate funding for hospitals to allow adequate staffing is nowhere to be seen.

---

1.   Aiken, LH, et al. Hospital nurse staffing and patient mortality, nurse burnout, and job dissatisfaction. *JAMA* 2002; 288:1987-93.

2.   The above study published in the *Journal of the American Medical Association* was the subject of a rather pointed editorial in the *New York Times* entitled "Dying for Lack of Nurses", October 25, 2002.

Many court challenges to ERISA have barely impacted its mandate. Huge lobbying efforts in Washington continue to make certain that the act remains intact and unmodified. One major lobbyist is The ERISA Industry Committee [3]. It appears to be backed by a number of major industry groups. Its credo is "Representing the Employee Benefits Interest of America's Largest Employers." I would redefine that goal as "Holding Down the Outrageous Cost of Benefits." This organization argues that workers and their families will ultimately bear the cost of expanded liability. It is true that expanded liability costs for HMOs and third-party benefit plan administrators will be passed along to employers and then to employees. Some of this pass-through will be in the form of higher premiums, and some might be in the form of higher costs of goods and services. The argument is made by the industry group that "defensive medicine," the ordering of extra medical tests and services for the sole purpose of avoiding legal liability, would become rampant if the exemptions under ERISA were repealed.

These arguments neglect the harsh reality that patients and their families bear the burden of delayed diagnosis and undertreatment of illness. The hard data to support the following idea does not yet exist: It is a nearly universal impression among all professionals to whom I have spoken that the quality of medical care continues downward under the inverted incentives of capitated care. Opportunities to prevent and treat disabling illness are being missed. Later in this book, I will discuss the applicability of a national medical database in collecting the necessary data on health outcomes to prove these points.

If there is one population of patients most negatively impacted by capitation, it is the elderly covered by Medicare. Capitated plans were introduced as an option for Medicare recipients, with the lure of such extra benefits as drug coverage and coverage for eyeglasses, benefits not available under regular Medicare Part A and Part B. When people get older and sicker, they consume a tremendous proportion of the total health care services. Various studies have shown something approaching one third of all health care expenditures occur in the last six months of life. This sick, elderly population needs the constant availability of medical help, in person or by phone. The "efficiency" promoted by capitated plans means that the primary doctor has an incentive not to see the patient, not to talk to the patient, and to delegate as much of the care as possible to nurses or other professionals. After all, the care has already been paid for at a small fixed monthly rate, and it is actually financially punitive to take care of the patients' needs. In my view, capitation leads to the destruction of the professional person,

---

3.   http://www.eric.org

and ultimately the destruction of the entire health care system. As I write this, many managed care companies are eliminating their senior care plans, in which Medicare pays the company a fixed amount per month per patient for all the care that might be required. As mentioned, the company in turn passes the financial risk of caring for illness onto a pool of doctors and hospitals. They provide all the care needed while bearing the financial risk if the utilization of services ends up costing more than the fixed rate per member provided by the contract with the management company. In California, numerous medical groups have been bankrupted by taking the financial risk of caring for capitated seniors. Yet, the traditional fee-for service type of care permitted under Medicare Part A and Part B has also been causing financial stress to the U.S. Treasury, so new methods of controlling costs have been deemed necessary by Medicare officials. I'll discuss some of these in the next chapter.

DRGs, Medicare Fee Freezes, and Microregulation

In 1984, the giant federal agency administering Medicare, the Health Care Financing Administration or HCFA[1] implemented its fixed fee per admission method of hospital reimbursement for patient services. In an elaborate scheme, hospital stays of patients with Medicare insurance coverage were lumped into one of 270 diagnostic categories, the "diagnosis related groups" or DRGs. Allowance was provided for certain "co-morbidities," (complicating factors in the illness), and the hospital was reimbursed at a low fixed rate for the care of the patient, regardless of the length of stay. Fixed payment, based on the "diagnosis related group" or DRG, of the patient's illness changed the landscape in a revolutionary fashion. The golden era of voluptuous Medicare payments for each day of a hospital stay, for each procedure, and for each supply or drug used were over. The fixed rate payment for a hospital stay provided by the DRG category often did not equal the actual cost of providing services to the patient. Hospital revenues plummeted. Over time, many hospitals closed or merged. Many institutions hired an army of consultants to help decide on the best closure or merger combinations to cope with the falling revenues. New strategies to reduce the length of hospital stay and to reduce hospital expenses in caring for patients were implemented.

The DRGs, with their fixed payment per admission, changed the way hospitals functioned for their acute inpatient services. However, certain services such as home care nursing and rehabilitation services initially were reimbursed under the old fee-for-service arrangement. Since patients were being booted out of the hospital "sicker and quicker," a compensatory increase in the availability of rehabilitation services and home health nursing services was envisioned by the HCFA as a means of taking care of patients who were not yet well enough for independent

---

1.   The agency name "Health Care Financing Administration" or HCFA was changed in 2001. The current name is "Centers for Medicare and Medicaid Services" or CMS.

living at home. Hospitals rushed to open or expand rehabilitation programs and home health agencies to share in the remaining Medicare fee-for-service dollars. Surprise! The utilization of inpatient rehabilitation and home health nursing services ballooned at a much greater rate than that anticipated. Eventually, these services were switched to a DRG fixed payment system, and the services tended to whither. As of this writing, inpatient rehabilitation services are being shrunken and closed, and the availability of home health services is in decline. The placement of last resort for patients unable to return home is the skilled-care nursing facility, the "nursing home," the institution in which most patients and their families hope never to have to spend time.

There is great variability in how much a given type of health care service is used, which is directly correlated to how well it is paid for. Inpatient rehabilitation services are an excellent example. Is rehabilitation necessary? Consider the patient admitted to the acute hospital with a stroke, paralyzed on one side and with a speech impediment. Let's say that improvement is slow, and he is unable to walk or care for personal needs after a number of days in the hospital. Improvement to the point of being independent can be accelerated with intensive physical therapy and speech therapy. The chance of returning to one's own residence is better than that for a patient kept inactive in bed. On the inpatient rehabilitation service, the involvement of family and caregivers is welcome, so patients who are not quite fully independent can return to their residence with confident help surrounding them. Transfer from the acute hospital to the inpatient rehabilitation service became common for Medicare patients disabled by an illness in the 1980s. The DRG fixed payment for the acute hospital stay put great financial pressure on the hospital to move the patient out as soon as feasible. But a patient who cannot walk or feed himself cannot go directly home. The rehabilitation units were burgeoning in number due to their favored Medicare reimbursement status. Many patients benefited from stays of up to several weeks in these hospital units. However, as of this writing, rehabilitation wards are shrinking and closing, now that the hospital gets a smaller fixed payment per patient for rehabilitation services. The cost of complying with the ever-expanding regulations regarding appropriateness of rehabilitation admission also consumes a large quantity of hospital resources. Reams of paper, or megabytes of digitized records, must be kept to justify each and every service rendered to each stroke patient. The hidden expense of this record keeping is immense. One now can walk the corridors of a hospital and its rehabilitation ward and see more staff charting at computer terminals than working with the patient at the bedside. The twenty-year cycle of expansion and contraction of rehabilitation programs is reaching its nadir, pushed down by the weight of regulation.

In the doctor's office, efforts in the 1990s to hold down costs by insurance companies and Medicare have produced a nightmare of additional paperwork and regulations. In the case of Medicare, lack of compliance with the paperwork requirements carries the threat of criminal penalties. There have been many complaints to Medicare and to Congress from physician organizations about the strangulation of patient care by paperwork and regulation. Medicare established a "Physician Regulatory Issues Team," directed by an M.D., to deal with the complaints. A November 26, 2001 update by the team director listed 25 issues most prominent in doctor complaints about difficulties with the paperwork. Seven regulatory issues received special recognition as particularly noxious. Among these was the paperwork required from the doctor for medical equipment such as canes and wheelchairs, for diabetic supplies for monitoring blood glucose, and for laboratory services. In simpler times, a doctor merely scribbled a prescription for needed supplies, hopefully legibly, on a prescription blank. The patient took this prescription to a supplier. If insurance reimbursed the patient for part or all of the cost of the item, that payment occurred without much effort on the part of the doctor or medical supplier. The insurer was an inert "third-party" to the transaction between the patient and the doctor, and between the patient and the supplier of medical products and services. Now, for Medicare patients, the physician is required to justify the "medical necessity" of goods and services. The forms are elaborate, often multipage, and confusing either by design or because the bureaucratic minds that created them think in a different language from the doctor.

In the case of orders for laboratory services, medical necessity must be justified by the doctor by providing five-digit codes for the diagnosis of the patient for each item of blood tests. There are thousands of five-digit codes, and only certain ones will justify a given lab test. When I think of thousands of doctors' offices, clinics, and emergency rooms, full of sick patients, and I consider the thousands of irrelevant hours of labor spent coding laboratory orders, I realize how a great health care system can be destroyed when a large centralized third-party payer makes the rules, be it Medicare or a private insurer. The bureaucrats initiated the coding requirements in the 1990s with the publicly stated goal of reducing unnecessary laboratory tests and saving billions of dollars. I can assure the bureaucrats that many more billions of dollars of time, labor, and paper are being wasted complying with the intricate rules for justifying each five-dollar blood test. The common tests like blood counts and blood chemistries, done by the tens of thousands each day in the United States using efficient automated equipment, each require many different forms, filled in by the doctor, the doctor's staff, the laboratory staff, and in part by the patient. The hidden cost of processing this paperwork dwarfs the expense of actually performing common automated blood tests. The dollars spent would be much better spent on patient care.

When the patient is covered under a capitated plan, that is, an HMO-type of coverage with prepaid pools of money each month for the primary physician, the hospital, the emergency room, and the laboratory, then the rules change. There is actually less paperwork, because there is no specific reimbursement for each service from an insurer. Reimbursement to the doctor or doctor group is based in part on the overall rate of utilization of laboratory tests. The more tests done for a capitated group of patients, the more the doctor is financially penalized. The implications are fairly obvious: The fewer tests that a physician orders for pools of capitated patients, the more money he or she makes. When he or she does order the simple blood tests, there is less paperwork than for patients with fee-for-service insurance, because, in effect, the doctor or the doctor's group is paying for the test rather than a third-party insurer. Are you confused? So are the patients, lab technicians, billing clerks, and doctors' office staff. Billing errors, coding errors, and reimbursement errors run through the system like water rushing down rapids. The turbulence created contributes nothing to helping patients. The best answer that policy makers can come up with is to collect more data, promulgate new regulations, and require more intricate paperwork to regulate the existing paperwork. If federal dollars are at stake, the "Paperwork Reduction Notice" Act goes into effect, requiring public hearings to gather data about the paperwork problem. I assume that generates still more paperwork.

It amazes me that the system of third-party payment for health care has gone through such dramatic shifts in the 30-year period I have been involved with it. Back in the era of *carte blanche* payment for almost everything, doctors were free to order lab tests without much regulation by outsiders. In addition, doctors often owned the laboratory facilities in which the tests were performed. Even small labs were profitable, and until Congress outlawed the practice, referral of patients to one's own facilities for testing was common and lucrative for the doctor. To summarize, lab testing now requires such a noxious level of paperwork that the paperwork itself is a disincentive to order marginally necessary tests. In the case of patients with HMO-type health plans, there may be additional financial disincentive to order *necessary* tests. We have gone from a system where too much testing was handsomely rewarded to one in which there is a modest amount of punishment just for doing one's professional work appropriately and heavy penalties for vigorous utilization of laboratory testing.

Medicare carefully regulates the fees for virtually all laboratory testing. For all Medicare patients, the laboratory must accept the Medicare payment as payment in full. Increasingly, other insurance companies use the Medicare fee schedule as the benchmark for reimbursement. The 5.4 percent fee reduction for Medicare services mandated by Congress for 2002 was welcome news to private insurers, since they could follow the Medicare lead and lower their rate of reimbursement. The latest reduction of 4.4 percent for 2003 has been justified by the U.S. Congress and the President as necessary during a time of budget deficits. There will likely be fewer testing facilities available and longer lines at the remaining ones as laboratories are closed or consolidated in the face of falling income.

In discussing the situation with pathologists, those M.D.s responsible for laboratory testing, it is amazing how the regulatory maze has altered this segment of the health care industry. Only large laboratories, running thousands of tests of each type with high-tech automated equipment, remain in operation. There are small "draw stations" where blood samples are taken from patients, but the specimens must be placed on ice and transported to the central processing facilities. Very common tests, like the automated complete blood count and the automated multichannel chemistry panel, actually can be run for less than a dollar per test if one considers only the cost of the chemical reagents used and the apportioned cost of the expensive automated equipment. But there are much higher costs in labor not directly required to produce the result of the lab test. A technician or assistant has to register the patients each time they appear at the lab, verify their insurance and identity, and produce bar-coded labels so that the blood specimens will be tested for the proper patient when they get to the central processing facility. (Have you ever wondered whether that lousy result on a blood cholesterol test actually belonged to someone else?) The order for the laboratory test has to contain the proper coding from the doctor's office to justify the test, and this has to be entered into the laboratory database in order to collect reimbursement later for performing the test. If a Medicare patient needs one test, namely a complete blood count, $12 of labor expense may be generated in registering the patient, drawing the blood, and processing the information that includes the results, the billing, and the regulatory paperwork. In my area, Medicare reimburses the laboratory $3.85 for performing an automated complete blood count.

In the short run, new paperwork and regulation reduce the cost of lab testing to third-party insurers like Medicare. I worry about massive hidden long-term costs, however. In the real world of caring for patients, there is not a black and white divider between necessary and unnecessary testing. Rather, there is a broad gray zone of somewhat necessary tests. For example, a patient taking a drug to lower cholesterol levels has a small risk of developing an inflammation in the liver. The earliest sign of this problem is seen in elevated values for several liver enzymes that are detectable on an automated blood chemistry panel. The doctor may order a hundred liver chemistry panels, one on each patient taking the medication, every six months, in order to detect the one patient with the rising liver enzymes who needs a change in drug therapy. There are substantial short-term savings in playing the odds, in not ordering the routine monitoring. Once in a while, a patient will show up with advanced liver and muscle inflammation not caught early by the blood testing. The marginal cost, that is, the additional overall expense of preventing such an event might be thousands of dollars of blood tests yielding normal results in hundreds of patients. Of course, the very occasional case of outright liver failure requiring liver transplantation can cost many more thousands of dollars. Is the liver blood chemistry every six months in each patient on cholesterol lowering drugs medically necessary? In the broad view of the best outcome for the whole population for the fewest dollars, maybe not. If your liver or my liver or your spouse's liver is at stake, the testing seems very necessary.

To be a professional is to make autonomous decisions based on training and experience and to bear the responsibility for the consequences. When you are no longer empowered to make decisions in this way, professionalism declines. The sense of self-worth and accomplishment that drives the doctor through the busy days and nights declines. In measurable and in intangible ways, the quality of professional services deteriorates. To be required to justify a simple everyday blood test for a patient with reams of paper slowly destroys the doctor, while generating thousands of new jobs in Medicare and its contractor insurance companies to generate and track all the paper or digitized information. None of the paper contributes to the care of the patient or an improvement in health. All the billing and coding to justify a simple lab test have an unspoken underlying motivation, to reduce the utilization of services and cut costs on this year's budget for health care. The incalculable costs of demoralized doctors, caring less, doing slipshod patient care, becoming angry and grumpy, is never taken into account by the bureaucrats in their federal offices.

Medicare claims a very low administrative overhead relative to the benefits provided by the program. Yet, the mammoth piles of regulations dwarf the imagination. The volume of forms and digitized information required to comply with the regulations creates warehouses full of paper and computer servers full of gigabytes of information. Human labor is required to generate these forms and digitized data. I have not seen an estimate of the actual total cost of compliance with the regulations created by Medicare and other insurers. It would be a very difficult figure to calculate accurately, since compliance costs are distributed into small parcels of the work day of myriad persons in the health care system. I would estimate that more than 20 percent of the dollars spent on health care in the United States goes directly or indirectly toward compliance with regulations. This money is wasted in the sense that it does not help sick people and may actually divert scarce resources, like nurses, from care.

To the doctor, there is a more insidious negative effect of the microregulation of each small clinical decision. Many paperwork requirements are backed by the threat of penalties including fines and imprisonment for errors or omissions. As the expression goes, "Sometimes when you are paranoid, there is really someone chasing you." Doctors are trained to be independent thinkers, taking control of serious and unstable health problems, and bearing the responsibility for what happens to the patient. To be successful in patient care, a doctor needs to have confidence in his ability to solve a problem, or to know when to seek expert consultation for assistance. When the doctor becomes preoccupied with the hassles of paperwork and compliance, it distracts from the focus on the patient. The lower level employees of third-party payers and regulatory agencies have much less training and knowledge than the M.D.s whose work they judge. Even doctors, who have long demonstrated belief in the "Iron Man Fantasy" of invincibility, get worn down by the hours of preoccupation with the rules of the bureaucracies.

In the "Iron Man Fantasy," one believes that all those other doctors running around the hospital are well-rested, joyously seeing patients and doing surgery 120 hours per week, sneaking in some quality time with the family, and not suffering from fatigue or burnout or worries about the paperwork. The competitive nature of people selected for the medical profession leads them to deny that their own human qualities of fatigue or depression are a problem. When the burden of microregulation and its hours of paperwork is added to a busy week, a destructive anger develops. The feeling of being disrespected by an invisible force capable of punishing you for submitting the wrong codes on a form eats away at the professional spirit. Performance suffers and becomes uneven. Fairly important patient care issues are neglected. Quality of care diminishes.

In discussing the situation with Medicare officials, I find a total preoccupation with the short-term problem of reducing costs and creating new regulations to achieve this goal. Complex schemes and sets of rules, each accompanied by forms and paperwork, are elaborated in increasing quantities. Some people in high positions are aware of the pain experienced by doctors and hospitals in the efforts to process the paperwork and comply with the myriad rules. But it seems to me that the process of creating new regulations runs independently of the original goals of the organization and is an end in itself for teams of administrators on the government payroll.

There was an era in which most doctors were independent, solo general practitioners. They had complete autonomy in their decision-making. They were respected for their years of training and experience, and they were most fortunate to know very intimately the patients whom they served. Patients did not have to change doctors every time their insurance plan changed. Doctors were free to care for anyone seeking their help. Record keeping was not a major issue, nor was malpractice liability, and the doctor could practically move a mountain without filling in a single form for the insurance company or an agency of the federal, state, or county government. Microregulation of every decision was still a long way in the future. I will attempt to describe that era in the next chapter.

The Rise and Fall of the GP Who Walked on Water

Those of us over 50 remember receiving a different kind of medical care in our early years. I refer to the golden age of the General Practitioner or "GP" in the United States. The stereotype of the GP was romanticized in television series like "Marcus Welby." The GP often lived in the town or neighborhood where he practiced. His office was part of the house in which he lived. Office hours were posted beneath his name on a "shingle" outside the entry to the waiting room. The waiting room was an unguarded entrance for public access, and, basically, most appointments to see the doctor were "walk-ins." Patients showed up during the hours for office services specified on the shingle and waited their turn to be seen. When not seeing patients in the office, the doctor was busy making house calls. A patient too sick to leave his or her residence would phone the doctor and ask for a house call. The doctor would show up, typically dressed in a flannel suit with a large black bag in hand, and ceremoniously be shown to the bedside. Well into the 1950s, office and home visits by the GP were paid for in cash and not covered by medical insurance. Medical insurance, when available, was of the "major medical and hospital" variety, to cover part of the cost of surgery and hospital stays. A typical fee for an office visit in the early 1950s was $5.00, and a house call was $8.00. (But it was the time when $10 purchased enough groceries for a family of four for a week).

To a young patient in 1950, the GP was a superhuman. When the parents were unable to fix an injury or health problem, the doctor was there to take care of it. When grandma was dying of cancer of the esophagus in a bed in the living room, there was Dr. Spivey with his black bag, making house calls early each morning and late each evening, sometimes dashing over in his Cadillac during lunch, injecting morphine from a big reusable glass syringe. Grandma stopped moaning immediately upon hearing his voice. By 2000, we have "comfort care" for end-of-life "home management" of patients dying of cancer, and we call it "hospice care." An M.D. is hardly to be seen in the hospice set-up. A team of nurses, aides, and social workers from the local Hospice organization implements the care, with an M.D. "medical director" signing off the paperwork in an office somewhere far from the patients. Medicare and many private insurance plans cover hospice services, and the paperwork related to each patient is thicker than several phone directories.

The neighborhood GP of 1950 was held in the highest esteem. "Dr. Spivey knows *everything.*" If you ran into Dr. Spivey at a social function or in some public place, it was difficult to look in his direction, since the light was too bright. Yet, he could keep you relaxed with "verbal anesthesia" alone while putting a couple of stitches in the nasty laceration on your leg you suffered from falling on a broken bottle. Many GPs delivered babies, and photos of their successes often wallpapered a hallway in their offices. They also did surgery or assisted in surgery at the local community hospital, set fractures, and took care of institutionalized patients in nursing facilities.

The GP made a comfortable living, though the hours were long, and sleep deprivation was a problem. Most GPs ran solo practices. Coverage for urgent cases might be arranged with nearby colleagues to allow a day off or a vacation with the family, but a significant proportion of solo practitioners were "workaholics," seeing patients day after day, week after week. Malpractice insurance was hardly needed. One retired GP told me that he first felt the need for malpractice insurance in the Chicago area in 1954, and the premium was $46 per year. Paperwork was also minimal. A patient's medical record often consisted of a 5" X 7" file card, on which was coded the dates of service, whether a fee was paid, and a brief scribble about the nature of the problem and medication given. Yet, the GP knew the details of the medical and personal history of several thousand patients of all ages. He "brought them into the world," as was the perception of delivery in the era of heavy sedation and little participation by the mother. He pronounced them dead, often in bed at home, or at the public place where they collapsed and expired of a heart attack. There were no paramedics and there was no CPR to attempt to revive people in cardiac arrest. There was just Dr. Spivey, grimly crouching over the still body on the ground, listening intently with a stethoscope and feeling for a pulse. After a minute, he looked up at the concerned circle of horrified people gathered around, and quietly said, "He's gone." Dr. Spivey methodically packed up his black bag, asked where there was a phone, and helped a relative call the undertaker who would transport the corpse to the funeral home. After a brief concerned offer of condolence and support to the spouse, hand on shoulder of the stunned and weeping family, he was gone, the Cadillac pulling away from the curb and disappearing.

What was the GP, and from what source came his perceived greatness? Why did he disappear, a phenomenon still mourned by older citizens today?

In the United States around 1900, medical education was in a shambles. Many doctors were regarded as charlatans and quacks. Some rural doctors also did veterinary work. In urban areas, prestige for medical men (and there were almost no women in the profession then) was restricted to the few talented surgeons available in a region who could safely get the patient through a complicated gallbladder surgery or radical mastectomy. There was sterile surgical technique, but no antibiotics, and little technology to help with problems considered routine a hundred years later. Care at the bedside for lesser problems involved the use of patent medicines, and often mixtures of opiates and laxatives were prescribed for myriad minor problems.

Reform of the system began with the Flexner Report of 1910[1]. The Carnegie Foundation, devoted to the improvement of education, sponsored this landmark study. A uniform medical school curriculum was proposed, with two years of basic science and two years of clinical clerkships on the wards of charity hospitals. Then came an intense year of the rotating internship, with several months in each major clinical area: obstetrics, pediatrics, surgery, and adult medicine. Following these five years of study and training, a young doctor usually was eager to find a niche as a GP. A few doctors went on to a rigorous three-year residency in general surgery or to specialized work in pathology or radiology. The reform to medical education and training brought by the Flexner Report altered the professional landscape for decades to come.

By the 1930s, there were significant numbers of well-trained GPs in the United States. There was also the Depression, with vast unemployment and social upheaval. GPs dutifully carried on in their communities, day and night, often caring for patients with little prospect of getting paid for the services. Medical care was often compensated for with produce or meat from the farm.

In the 1940s more than half the GP population was drafted for military service during World War II. Those remaining in their communities were hard pressed to keep up with the volume of work, caring for the patients of colleagues in military service. After the war ended, the United States entered what we can look back upon as the Golden Age of the General Practitioner. The authority and autonomy of the GP was absolute. He stood at the pinnacle of social prestige in the community, and income was high relative to the rest of the population.

---

1.   Abraham Flexner, *Medical Education in the United States and Canada*, New York: Carnegie Foundation for the Advancement of Teaching, 1910

Marjorie Spradling lives near San Francisco, but was born and raised in Nebraska. She recently spent time with me reminiscing about the career of her rural General Practitioner father, Dr. Leslie Earl Sauer. "Doc," as everyone called him, practiced in Tekamah, Nebraska from 1925 until 1974. As a high school student, Marjorie assisted her father with running the office. She remembers folding gauze bandages, wrapping them in cloth, and placing them in a steam sterilizer. She mailed bills and assisted at tonsillectomies done in the office.

Doc was highly regarded around the area, treated with reverence, the GP who walked on water. He delivered somewhat more than 2500 babies during his career. He worked every day, even when he had a partner. Marjorie remembers only one extended vacation of two-and-a-half weeks, when the family traveled to the New York World's Fair in 1939. "Doc" would take hunting and fishing trips with friends for a few days. His wife went on vacations with her friends, since her husband was usually working.

There were morning and afternoon office hours and late afternoon and evening house calls. An office visit cost $4 in the 1940s. Many people were unable to pay. Some left chickens or corn on the front seat of Doc's car in lieu of cash. By the way, the car was never locked, and the large black bag that sat on the front seat was stocked with many drugs, including morphine.

Marjorie describes her father as compassionate, factual, and honest. He had his human failings as well, tossing the telephone when he was angry, and tending to be a bit sadistic when caring for his own family. He smoked cigarettes, eventually having small strokes, but living to age 90.

In Tekamah, Nebraska, Doc shared prestigious status with two other types of professionals in town, lawyers and bankers. He was able to afford a comfortable but not extravagant lifestyle for his family, with hired household help and automobiles. He enjoyed woodworking as a hobby, having been born to a carpenter father, and was able to spend a small amount of time in his woodshop.

Numerous patients and friends have related stories to me of the GP of their youth. One friend, Fred Arvidson, describes his father-in-law, a physician in rural Illinois, as "the only physician in a 40 mile radius in a rural farming area." In September, on the way home from evening hospital rounds, he would pull over to the side of a road and hunt pheasant in a farmer's field "reserved" for him. When he died, school was closed for a day so a memorial service could be held in the high school gymnasium. He had delivered most of the kids in the school." Many idolized the doctor who cared for them as a child, and some were inspired to a career in medicine or nursing by that individual's accomplishments. There is also a sense of lament that "they don't make them like they used to." Even people who have benefited from heart surgery or neurosurgery done by an excellent specialist in recent years look back more fondly to the memories of the GP of their earlier years. That doctor delivered them, saw them as sick children, took out their tonsils (whether necessary or not), and seemed to be available in person or by phone at any hour.

This type of care hardly exists anymore. In the present, there is too much to know to be proficient in handling all types of medical problems in people of all ages. No one will carry morphine in a big black bag stowed in his or her unlocked automobile. In addition, the paperwork required by federal and state regulatory agencies to stock the morphine and administer it makes the solo doctor house call much less useful for patients in pain. Newer agents which do not require injection are dispensed by an elaborate team of nurses, pharmacists and technicians in each hospice program, so the friendly GP is not the comforting figure at the bedside of people dying at home.

Our elaborate system of medical emergency response has rendered obsolete the image of the GP dashing off with the big black bag to the scene of an accident or heart attack. Now, specially trained emergency medical technicians do the appropriate first steps, stabilize the sick or injured patient, and haul them to the emergency room, that booming medical institution which I will discuss later. In some states, it has become illegal for a bystander M.D. to help paramedics at the scene of an accident or sudden illness. The professional role of caregiver in a life-threatening situation has been abdicated.

Actually, the death knell for the GP was already sounding in the 1960s. According to the American Board of Family Practice, by 1964 the percentage of medical school graduates going into general practice had fallen to 19 percent. The age of specialization had begun, and the volume of knowledge was too great for a generalist to assimilate in a one-year of rotating internship after medical school. A new specialty of family practice was established in 1969, with a three-year residency training program following the four years of medical school. The goal was to continue the tradition of the General Practitioner, providing comprehensive, personal, and family care. But the specialty has never really fulfilled its potential to be the source of primary care doctors for the majority of the population. The negative forces impacting the medical profession strike hardest at the front line troops in the field.

Specialization and Subspecialization: Something Gained and Something Lost

With the arrival of health insurance for a large portion of the population in the 1950s and 1960s, funds were available for teaching hospitals and training programs for doctors. In fact, Medicare had a special subsidy for care in a teaching hospital in its earlier years. The expansion of technology led to the need for new types of expert doctors, specially trained to use new methods to make people well. Thus began the decline of the GP and many of the benefits of the friendly neighborhood doctor who knew everyone in the family.

The original four clinical specialties had been around since before the days of the Flexner Report of 1910 which standardized the rotating internship to include these areas in the training of new medical school graduates. They were obstetrics and gynecology to care for women of childbearing age and their deliveries, pediatrics for children, internal medicine (more accurately described as adult medicine), and surgery. When an adult seen by a GP had a complicated heart problem, an internist would be consulted to further define the problem and see what could be done to treat it. A child with nephritis, an inflammation of the kidneys, might have been sent by the GP to a pediatrician affiliated with a teaching hospital. But the GP remained the center of care as far as the patient and family were concerned.

Suddenly, there was new technology. By the 1960s, taking care of a patient with heart disease no longer meant listening to a murmur with a stethoscope and administering digitalis. Now there were "invasive" techniques, heart catheterization and angiography. Thin plastic tubes called catheters could be threaded via a large blood vessel in the leg. Through the catheter, a dye could be squirted to make the blood flow through the heart and coronary arteries visible on X-ray. The coronary angiogram is the movie made of the flow of blood inside the heart and through its arteries. Performing this procedure was certainly beyond the expertise of the GP and even beyond the expertise of the first line of referral, the

35

internist. The subspecialty of cardiology became an important area of clinical care, with the widespread prevalence of heart disease and the new technology that promised curative treatment. To become proficient at what is called "invasive cardiology" requires at least five years of training beyond medical school, three in a residency in internal medicine and two years of postdoctoral fellowship in cardiology to learn the new angiography procedures. These days, there may be additional years of training to learn the techniques of opening clogged coronary arteries with balloons and new techniques such as treating the arteries with radioactive inserts so they will not clog up again.

The new procedures are very expensive and contribute greatly to the rise in the cost of health care. Unfortunately, they rarely fulfill the hope of the 1960s, that given enough technology, a disease could be completely cured. We are still experiencing epidemic atherosclerosis in the United States, the clogging of arteries with cholesterol-laden crud which ultimately kills nearly half of us. Opening up a totally clogged or nearly clogged blood vessel with the new techniques is only a stop-gap to prevent a catastrophe like a fatal heart attack caused by closure of that blood vessel. It does not address the problem that the process of atherosclerosis is continuing in blood vessels all over the body. Other blood vessels can slowly clog, leading to stroke, gangrene of a foot, kidney failure, or blindness, even after fixing of the blockage in the coronary artery. Expensive medication, taken daily, is needed to help slow the disease process. So, the patient needs the continued care of the cardiologist to see if the unclogged artery in the heart stays open and to try to slow the clogging of other arteries with medication. Periodic stress tests are done to check heart function. Despite the success of the new procedures, the patient is still a heart patient seeing the cardiologist on a regular basis. Should the patient ask the cardiologist during an office visit for some help with a painful hemorrhoid, the cardiologist will often say something like "see your family doctor or internist, since I don't take care of hemorrhoids." Some cardiologists might say, "It's been years since I've treated hemorrhoids; I'm a heart specialist. I wouldn't know what to do for this condition." In some cases, the cardiologist may bypass the primary doctor of the patient and send the patient for consultation with a surgical subspecialist, a colorectal surgeon, who is expert at treating hemorrhoids.

Given the expense and time delays of seeing different experts for each part of the body, the modern scenario of subspecialization may seem a bit trying to the patient. Older people will glorify the past age of the neighborhood GP, who did "everything." Of course, there was much less treatment available in 1950, and one doctor really was able to do nearly everything for all patients. Patients having a heart attack were put at absolute bedrest for four weeks, and more than half died. The GP was there to pronounce death but had few tools to prevent it.

Another problem with subspecialization is the occurrence of duplication of services and errors of omission. Different specialists may order the same tests on the same patient for somewhat different reasons. We do not have a master system to track this unnecessary duplication, and I have seen it involve expensive imaging studies like computed tomography (CT) scans and magnetic resonance (MR) scans, tests costing many hundreds of dollars. There is no standardized system of communication among doctors for a large portion of the patient population, and no one central repository of the essential data on the patient. An involved primary care physician, assuming a central and strong role in a patient's care, can help coordinate the fragmented specialty and subspecialty interventions, but a doctor playing such a role is increasingly rare.

Much subspecialty care is given at a hospital or outpatient surgery center, since the equipment and personnel required to perform high-tech procedures exceed what is financially plausible for a single doctor's office. This adds another bewildering dimension of care for the patient. A large, impersonal clinic setting is much less comfortable to the patient than a friendly and familiar office.

Also contributing to the disinterest in the patient and demoralization of the doctor is the rise of managed care. In capitated plans, the patient is no longer a human being, but is a commodity, a "covered life." The fiscal goal for the doctors is to collect as many covered lives as possible, and then limit access to care as much as possible. In subtle and not so subtle ways, the patient is made to feel like an unwelcome guest. Many problems are not taken care of until they become an emergency. Even the simple problems of a patient tend to be shunted elsewhere, as described in the following chapter.

"Go to the Emergency Room!"

There is no longer easy access to the neighborhood general practitioner for the troublesome sore throat, bellyache, or sore elbow. Despite all the rhetoric in recent years about efficiency of health care delivery in large HMOs and all the discussion of overutilization of medical services, most people seeking care urgently have simple problems that are not expensive to deal with. The simple, accessible, friendly home cottage industry of the local GP actually was a very efficient form of health care service. The doctor was in the town or neighborhood. He would come to you with a well-stocked gear bag if you could not get to him.

We are in a new age of health care in which an increasing number of patients can only get urgent, same-day service if they go to an emergency room. One of the perverse consequences of capitated health plans, the HMOs, is that many of them provide financial incentive for the doctor not to see a sick patient expeditiously. As is the jargon in the trade, there may be, in effect, a fiscal incentive to "turf" the patient with the minor problem to the emergency room.

Consider a typical scenario: Mrs. Jones is a healthy 38 year old woman whose health insurance is the California Mega Health Plan. She is actually unaware that she is a capitated patient in an HMO. The glossy brochure listing all the services covered by a $15 co-payment per visit seemed wonderful relative to the comparatively low premium. She has received routine "well-woman" exams in a family practice group office near her home. The care was a bit impersonal, but satisfactory. Now, Mrs. Jones has a terrible sore throat and she is in the eighth day of her illness. She is having considerable pain with swallowing. She calls the family practice office. First, she hears a recorded message, "If this is an emergency, please hang up and dial 9-1-1. Otherwise, listen carefully to the following six menu choices. Push the pound key if you would like to start this message again." Choice number five is the option of transfer to a real, live person. Mrs. Jones pushes five, and hears a recording apologizing that the real live person is "either away from my desk or helping another patient." Mrs. Jones is an experienced citizen of the twenty first century, so she reads a magazine while waiting on hold and listening to big band music mixed with static.

"You have been seen here before, right?" asks the phone receptionist after a twenty minute wait on hold.

Mrs. Jones replies foggily, "Yes, I saw Dr. Smith and his nurse practitioner last year."

"Let me look you up in the computer." Pause. "Do you still have California Mega Health Plan?"

"Yes."

"Well, I'm sorry, Dr. Smith is at a meeting this morning, and all the other doctors have full appointments today and tomorrow."

"But I can't swallow!"

"Well, maybe you'd better go to the emergency room!"

"Uh, OK."

Mrs. Jones goes to the Emergency Room at the local community hospital near her home, part of a "participating Health System" listed in her HMO brochure. She is surprised to find it very crowded on a weekday morning. At the registration desk, a triage nurse asks her a few questions about her problem, determines that it is not life threatening, and asks her to wait in the waiting area. Four hours later, she is ushered into an examining cubicle by another nurse, told to put on a paper gown, and the nurse checks her temperature and blood pressure and takes a brief history. There is commotion outside the cubicle, with footsteps running down the corridor. "There's another code in number three!" she hears from around the corner.

Another hour goes by, and a slightly harried and disheveled doctor comes into the examining cubicle. "Hi, I'm Dr. Gorkney, why are you here today?" Mrs. Jones describes her problem once again. The doctor examines her cursorily, noting her bright red throat but clear lungs and otherwise healthy history and appearance. "You may have a strep throat. I would like to order a throat culture and start you on some antibiotics." A nurse comes in and swabs Mrs. Jones' throat for a strep culture, asks her if she'd like to get her antibiotic at the hospital pharmacy, and starts the paperwork for discharge from the emergency room.

Seven hours have passed since Mrs. Jones first called the family practice office about her sore throat. She is now home with a bottle of antibiotic capsules. There is an elaborate patient education printout with all the potential side effects listed. She has several pieces of paper, one of which is the post-emergency room instruction sheet, telling her she has been treated for "pharyngitis, rule out streptococcal pharyngitis," and instructing her to return to the emergency room if she develops difficulty breathing.

Back in the billing office of the Health System that operates the hospital, the nominal charges for Mrs. Jones' emergency room encounter are being posted at a computer terminal. There is a $650 charge for use of the emergency room, a $225 charge for comprehensive emergency room assessment by the M.D., and a $45 charge for streptococcal throat screening culture. There is also a $52 charge from the hospital pharmacy for the antibiotic. I use the term "nominal charges" because they are for bookkeeping and financial planning purposes only. Since Mrs. Jones is a capitated patient in an HMO, actual reimbursement to the hospital is a fixed sum per month. The hospital might get something like $90 per month for all the care that might be required by Mrs. Jones, even for the very unlikely event that she would require heart bypass surgery. The patient who is uninsured or self-insured will receive a bill for the entire $972 worth of services listed above. In the case of Mrs. Jones, the computer cranks out a bill to her of $112, of which $60 is the co-payment required of the patient for an emergency room visit, and $52 for the antibiotic. Of the $90 received from California Mega Health Plan by the hospital that month for Mrs. Jones's care, a small portion of it is allocated to the group of emergency medicine doctors who staff the emergency room under contract with the Health System. They might receive ten cents per member per month to provide all necessary emergency room care.

If you are lost in these numbers, you are not alone! The key points are that Mrs. Jones used up most of a day getting medical care for a troublesome sore throat, possibly strep, and generated a bill of nominally $972 for medical services via the emergency room. She will owe $112 for this encounter. The hospital will collect $90 per month for Mrs. Jones from Mega Health Plan, keeping more of it if Mrs. Jones uses fewer hospital services. The nominal charge of $225 for the emergency room physician is used to calculate his share of the capitation payments that are apportioned each month to the emergency medicine doctor group by the hospital. In reality, he will earn approximately $18 for his encounter with Mrs. Jones.

Remember old Dr. Spivey, the neighborhood GP? In the 1950s, Mrs. Jones would have gone to his waiting room without an appointment and paid $5 cash for an office visit and $3 for a shot of penicillin. She would have been well known to Dr. Spivey, who would not have been accustomed to seeing this healthy woman very often and would understand her concern about the swallowing difficulty and the persistence of the symptoms. The therapeutic effect of a doctor knowing the patient, being available, and being concerned is diluted away in the setting of the emergency room. This is not to say that there is not empathetic care in the emergency room. Thousands of dedicated nurses and other staff who work in that department give it their best each shift. But during peak periods when clusters of critically ill patients arrive, it is impossible to give the extra time and care to each patient and his or her family. This is an era of tight hospital budgets, and staffing in the emergency room is not lavish. It is also the time of a nursing shortage, and available positions for nurses may go unfilled.

Among the patients visiting the emergency room, many are like Mrs. Jones. They have an urgent problem with distressing symptoms, but the illness is not life threatening. The lack of availability of care in a timely fashion in a doctor's office leads the patient to the emergency room for help, because there is no other option. In discussing this problem with experienced emergency room (ER) nurses, it is clear that a majority of patients filling the emergency rooms these days do not have a dire illness. Patients seeking ER care can be stratified into three categories: Those with life or limb threatening illness or injury, 20 percent; those with urgent, uncomfortable symptoms who need help within hours to relieve symptoms, 60 percent; those with non-urgent problems of a mild or chronic nature, 20 percent. Mrs. Jones' bad and persistent sore throat falls into the middle category, as do a majority of illnesses seen in the ER.

At the community hospital where I spent so many hours, the patient load and intensity of illness were variable and often unpredictable. As the volume of ER patients increased, the periods during which the emergency department turned into a "zoo" increased in frequency and duration. What is meant in the trade by the term "zoo?" Well, consider a relaxed time in the emergency department. There are patients in only six of the thirteen examining cubicles. Let's say that one patient is wired to a heart monitor, having come in by ambulance with what appears to be a stable, twelve hour old heart attack. The patient is getting some tests, is being seen by the cardiologist, and will shortly be transported up to the cardiac care unit on a portable monitor, with stable vital signs. Two patients have uncomplicated lacerations requiring suturing by the emergency room doctor. One patient has a fever of 103 and diarrhea. A child is wheezing, but without any major breathing difficulty. And an elderly patient fell down, has a pelvic fracture not requiring surgery, and will be admitted for observation, pain control, and placement (probably in a nursing facility).

What is a "zoo?" I will describe it, but you have to be involved in it to appreciate the intensity. All thirteen gurneys[1] are filled in the exam cubicles, and several

---

1. A gurney is defined by the American Heritage Dictionary® as a metal stretcher with wheeled legs, used for transporting patients, probably after J. Theodore Gurney, American inventor who patented a type of wheeled horse-drawn cab in 1883.

gurneys line the hallways. Out in the waiting area, all chairs are filled, and some patients are standing outside the doors, planning on a long wait. In one cubicle, there is a dead eight month old infant, apparently a case of Sudden Infant Death Syndrome (SIDS). One of the ER doctors and the hospital chaplain are standing in the room with the distraught parents, and now a pair of wailing grandparents has been brought in. In another cubicle, there is a combative drunk with a head laceration. A police officer is standing over him. He is restrained, tied to the side-erails of the gurney with leather cuffs, but he is writhing and cursing in a loud voice. Several infants are crying in other rooms, with an occasional piercing shriek as they are examined. Several ambulances arrive at the ambulance dock, and there are no spaces in which to put their cargo, so more guerneys fill the hall outside the treatment area. A patient with chest pain who staggered in on foot 10 minutes ago and was placed on a monitor now goes into cardiac arrest, and a Code Blue is called, causing more commotion…

Scenes like this are repeated over and over in all types of hospitals across the country each day. In some crowded urban emergency rooms, the staff will say, "It is always a zoo." Yet, 80 percent of patients seen in the emergency room do not have a life-threatening illness. These are the patients who do not have an available primary care doctor who is able to see them quickly with same day service. It is a growing population, as the number of doctors on the front lines declines due to all the forces described in this book.

There is a solution. If it is financially viable to take care of patients in an office, they will be taken care of in the office. Remember that roughly 80 percent of patients seen in the emergency room have a non-critical problem. The majority of these patients do not require the expensive facilities of the hospital to get care and relief. The services that have a nominal cost of $800 to $1000 in the emergency department cost $80 to $100 in the doctor's office. I use the term "nominal" because few patients pay these charges. There is a large statutory reduction in fees for Medicare and Medicaid patients, for the latter to a small fraction of the charges. There are contractual deep discounts by private insurers. And if the patient is capitated, there is a small co-payment by the patient as the only incentive to the doctor to see the patient in the office. We need to restore office care by paying a bounty per patient seen in the office urgently. We need to pay doctors enough for urgent office care to make them fight to see patients with urgent problems, rather than to tell them to go to the emergency room. Doctors are no longer in control of their fees, but those who control the fees would produce tremendous savings to the entire health care system by supporting office care with higher fees and a bounty for same-day service of urgent problems.

Drugs: The Best Outcomes Money Can Buy

"Outcome analysis" is a term that has come into wide use in recent years in the health care profession. We hope that our new medical technologies will provide better outcomes, that is, cure disease with minimal side effects. We hope to do the most good for the greatest number of people while causing the least harm. We have left behind the era of the paternalistic general practitioner whose knowledge was based on experience and whose judgment was regarded as infallible. This is the new era of seeking certainty through clinical studies and the collection and analysis of data. The term "evidence-based medicine" has become popular to describe scientifically verified medical treatment, based on an evaluation of the level of success ("outcome") of available approaches to treatment. The treatment of many common diseases has been distilled into "treatment algorithms," cookbook-style listings of diagnostic and treatment procedures. Available in medical specialty journals and on-line, these "gold standards" assure a certain uniformity to and minimum standard of patient care, particularly when physician-extenders like nurse practitioners are involved in the direct care of the patient. "Evidence-based medicine" is supposed to be the best medicine. The medical science that doctors follow and in which patients place their faith is assumed to be objective and unbiased. However, in regard to pharmaceuticals, those who measure the effects of new medicines on disease are often the companies that produce them or individuals who depend on the producers for funding; instead of being completely impartial, they are highly vested in the "outcomes" of the analyses.

In recent years, the companies that develop, manufacture, and market new drugs and technologies have played an ever-expanding role in this success of medicines as treatments. The pharmaceutical industry is a major economic and political force in the United States. Through strong lobbying efforts in Washington, it has largely escaped the price regulation seen in many developed nations in the world and in other areas of the health care system in the United States. The Pharmaceutical Research and Manufacturers of America (PhRMA) is one of the largest lobbying organizations in the Capitol. It provides millions of dollars of campaign contributions to Republicans and Democrats alike, while its member corporations invest billions of dollars annually in the research and development of new drugs. A significant portion of the dollars for human research now comes from the pharmaceutical manufacturers, including the funding for many of the studies performed in doctors' offices and at independent university medical centers.

Pharmaceutical companies were free to market drugs as they chose until the infamous thalidomide tragedy of the late 1950s. Use of this medication during pregnancy caused severe birth defects, with shortened or absent limbs. Some babies were born with their hands growing directly out of their shoulders. This tragedy was the stimulus for the passage of the Food, Drug, and Cosmetic Act of 1961, mandating the Food and Drug Administration (FDA) to determine the "safety and efficacy" of each new drug brought to market and to implement standards for product labeling. Each new drug is now taken through a four-phase study: First phase testing is done to look for toxicity in animals and the second phase in healthy human paid volunteers to screen for adverse effects on the organs of well people. Third, there is testing for effectiveness in sick patients according to a controlled, double-blinded protocol, and then, lastly, a new drug is subjected to a post-marketing surveillance phase to look for other side effects with actual use in the real world. Obtaining FDA approval for a new drug is an elaborate process that can take five years or longer. The cost of bringing a new drug to market can exceed $800 million. The pharmaceutical companies aim to recoup this expense while the new, branded agents are protected by patent, at prices far greater than those for older generic drugs with expired patents. Once a successful drug's patent expires, there are usually several manufacturers lined up for approval by the FDA to produce the unbranded generic version of the medication, and the price may fall to 10 percent of that of the branded version.

According to the pharmaceutical manufacturers, the high cost of new medications is justified by the high costs of research and development. Long-term success of the company depends upon having a flow of potential new blockbusters in the pipeline. According to PhRMA[1], there are 371 biotechnology medicines in testing, 800 medicines for the diseases of aging, and nearly 200 for diseases of children. The need for human subjects for clinical trials of new drugs, and the need for funds at university medical centers, has led to a partnering of academic physicians at teaching hospitals and the pharmaceutical industry. Increasingly,

---

1.   http://www.phrma.org/whoweare/presscorner/01.11.2002.603.cfm

the economic survival of the medical faculty in the academic medical realm depends upon obtaining research grants from drug companies to investigate new medications in sick patients. Twenty years ago, a greater proportion of research funding came from government agencies. Over the past two decades, as the federal government has attempted to put a lid on health care expenditures, there has been a decrease in the proportion of total medical research spending financed by government grants, compared to that provided by industry. There are still more than $10 billion per year funded by the National Institutes of Health, an important source of funding for diseases like cancer, coronary disease, and Alzheimer's disease. But funding by industry has grown to double that amount, and this now comprises the majority of all money spent on medical research.

There are hidden forms of bias in the private sponsorship of research. The drugs selected for testing tend to be those with potentially large markets. Many fewer dollars are spent researching agents with small market potential, such as those for rare diseases. Additionally, if a researcher produces data that show the safety and efficacy of an investigational new drug, such an outcome fulfills the goals of the sponsoring pharmaceutical company to move a potential new agent through the pipeline. On the surface, the scientific method seems to eliminate any bias. But the data may be manipulated. For example, the study design may allow for the disqualification of data from a patient in a study if certain seemingly irrelevant adverse events occur. If a patient is dropped from the study midcourse because of a sudden attack of appendicitis, the data from that patient may be excluded from the study results. Yet, drugs cause occasional very bizarre adverse events. We tend to ignore these as irrelevant until they occur multiple times, but in the study population of several hundred patients, they may only appear once or twice. Another example is the use of a study to compare the new agent to an older, already obsolete generic drug, rather than a newer, better drug in the same category produced by a different pharmaceutical company. The FDA, in its requirement for safety and efficacy, does not mandate that comparison be made to any particular drug used to treat the same disease. Merely demonstrating superiority to a very old medication and demonstrating safety will fulfill the licensing requirements.

It is just this kind of subtle manipulation that allows biased but supposedly objective results to be generated, ultimately leading to the approval of an expensive new agent with minimal advantages over cheaper older drugs, or with serious underreported adverse effects. The drugs selected for testing tend to be those with potentially large markets. Many new, expensive drugs that are brought to market are "me-too" drugs, similar to best-sellers already on the market, with sufficient minor changes in the chemistry of the drug molecules to make them patentable. These agents tend to belong to categories for which there is a huge market, such as drugs used to treat chronic conditions like hypertension, elevated cholesterol, or diabetes.

Phase Four, or post-marketing surveillance studies, as well as Phase Three, or trials of a drug on ill but non-hospitalized patients, have been moved from university hospitals in recent years. Private physicians' offices around the U.S. are now a favored venue for drug studies, since many of the promising new agents are for patients who are in the community, not in the hospital, and requiring treatment for a chronic condition such as those mentioned above. A doctor or group of doctors, lured by the high reimbursements from the pharmaceutical companies for performing the studies, may find that a substantial proportion of practice earnings can be derived from participation in drug research. Often, a designated nurse-research coordinator hired by the doctors performs most of the data collection. There are many safeguards in place to protect the patients, including elaborate "informed-consent" paperwork. Patients are told of all the potential side effects of an investigational agent and of the fact that neither they nor the staff will know whether they are receiving the experimental drug or a placebo. However, experts familiar with the process tell me that patients who become subjects in a study run by "their doctor" maintain the attitude that "the doctor has me on a new drug that is going to help me." At least 30 percent of the beneficial effect of a drug used to treat a troubling symptom is the placebo effect. Placebos, sugar pills resembling an expensive prescribed medication, give substantial relief of pain, for example. It is human psychology to want to believe in the positive effect of a healing agent. "Ya gotta believe" is a well-known part of the art of medicine. Patients, when convinced that a therapeutic intervention will help them, do better than patients who feel hopeless about a treatment. Given the powerful placebo effect of any intervention, I wonder how this influences the results of a study. Will subject patients report fewer side effects while in a research protocol performed in this fashion from their own doctor's office? Even if the patient is recruited for the study via a newspaper or radio advertisement, the private office venue for the study makes it seem as though an omnipotent personal doctor is performing a therapeutic manipulation on their behalf with a potentially miraculous new drug specific to their health problem.

In office-based studies, the doctor is being compensated based on the quantity of patient data submitted. The more subjects that complete the study, the greater the payment to the M.D. Does this provide an incentive to "cook the data" and produce complete data sets for patients who may not have actually completed the study? The academic journals are filled with recent reports of studies the conclusions of which have been retracted due to the discovery of forged results, where the researcher created data to support a positive outcome for a drug or medical procedure. The poor quality of medical research was the subject of a recent paper[2] in which the author pointed out the rampant methodological errors in human research. A potentially more onerous trend was recently reported[3]. Several large advertising firms have quietly purchased companies that perform clinical trials of experimental drugs. These companies are contractors for the major pharmaceutical houses, and carry out the logistics of running the human studies. The ad agencies have built a multi-billion dollar business promoting drugs to consumers. They are now expanding the uses of new and expensive drugs by running studies to "prove" the efficacy of new treatments, an outcome strongly in their fiscal interest.

Another trend of questionable long-term effect is the movement of the site of medical research offshore. Both animal and human studies of drugs are now so highly regulated, with such voluminous recordkeeping requirements, that pharmaceutical companies contract with researchers in foreign countries to do biomedical research there. One director of clinical research for a pharmaceutical company recently told me that the volume of paperwork for each rat used in pre-clinical studies in the U.S. now fills a file cabinet drawer, much of it to provide documentation for government inspectors of the humane handling of the animal. It has become much less expensive to do the research abroad. What additional confounding variables are introduced into the research by doing it in another country?

It is not uncommon for the FDA to order the withdrawal of a previously approved and seemingly successful drug from the market following reports of adverse reactions and death. In 2001, Bayer Pharmaceuticals had to withdraw its star cholesterol-lowering drug, Baycol®, because an unexpectedly large number of patients developed liver damage while taking the medication. Was the problem evident in the data presented to the FDA that led to the approval of Baycol® for marketing? Probably not. However, liver and muscle inflammation are potential side effects for this entire class of cholesterol-lowering medications. But one can speculate as to subtle biases that were a part of the data collection in Phase Three studies of the drug. Were there conflicts of interest, such as researchers highly

---

2.   Altman, DG. Poor-quality medical research. What can journals do? *JAMA* 2002;287:2765-67.

3.   Petersen, M. Madison Ave. plays growing role in drug research. *NY Times*, November 22, 2002

dependent upon their financial relationship with Bayer? Ultimately "outcome analysis" in the form of federally mandated post-marketing surveillance revealed the true frequency of severe side effects from the medication. The best "evidence-based medicine" was for Bayer to withdraw Baycol® from the market even before any official action by the U.S. FDA.

Unfortunately it is not only the research into medicines that is tainted by the funding source-beneficiary relationship. In a recently published study in the Journal of the American Medical Association[4], increasing contact was reported between authors of clinical practice guidelines and the pharmaceutical industry. What are clinical practice guidelines? These are the published summaries, the "treatment algorithms" mentioned at the outset of this chapter, by expert clinicians that attempt to synthesize recent research into recommendations for practice. Clinical practice guidelines have become very important in recent years, providing direction for the application of new technology to everyday clinical situations. They also become the standard of care in the event that the quality of a patient's care is brought under scrutiny, such as in malpractice litigation. The journal study showed that 87 percent of authors of clinical guidelines had had some form of interaction with the pharmaceutical industry. 58 percent had received some form of financial support to perform research and 38 percent had served as employees or consultants for a pharmaceutical company. Perhaps most disturbing is the findings that 59 percent of the authors of clinical guidelines had relationships with companies whose drugs were considered in the guidelines they authored. Presently, the financial conflicts of interest between the authors of clinical guidelines and the pharmaceutical companies who fund them are not disclosed in the published summaries of the guidelines, which are widely disseminated in print and electronically. Increasingly, as medical records and medical information become computerized, doctors and other health care providers have access to published guidelines at a terminal near the patient. These guidelines tend to be highly regarded as the best consensus of opinion on treatment, even as infallible. The published guidelines recommending the use of new and expensive drugs must be reevaluated in light of the severe conflicts of interest present in their creation.

One blood-clot-dissolving agent, tissue plasminogen activator or TPA, has been found useful in certain patients who are in the process of having a stroke. Most strokes occur when a blood clot forms in one of the small blood vessels in the brain; often, the clot occurs in a vessel narrowed by atherosclerosis, or hard-

---

4.   http://jama.ama-assn.org/issues/v287n5/abs/joc11772.html

ening of the arteries. An injection of TPA costs several thousand dollars and must be given within a few hours of the onset of the symptoms of the stroke to benefit the patient. A side effect of this potent blood thinner is hemorrhage into the brain, which carries a 50 percent fatality rate. The trade-off for the expense of the injected blood thinner and the risk of hemorrhage is a moderate improvement in outcome, that is, a reduction in the degree of paralysis from the stroke. Some doctors question whether the use of TPA is worthwhile at all. However, leading organizations, like the American Heart Association, have endorsed its use. The Heart Association has also developed a public education campaign to get people to the hospital at the earliest sign of stroke so that the medication can be given in a timely fashion. A special committee has published clinical guidelines for doctors for the use of TPA in recent-onset stroke. Use of this agent has therefore become the community standard in the emergency room. How much of the decision to endorse this drug is based on the recommendation of doctors who receive research money from the drug's manufacturer? When those who define policy are sponsored by the makers of expensive new agents, we risk decisions based on marginal evidence that does not weigh all the effects of the drug. We are biased toward celebrating the occasional spectacular "save" of a patient with a stroke by the injectable blood thinner and tend to ignore those in whom the stroke is made worse by a brain hemorrhage and who end up permanently disabled. Or, in other words, we have not given adequate numerical weight to the misery of a long-term vegetative state versus the slight improvement in successfully treated stroke victims, yielding "evidence-based medicine" more in keeping with the need to market the blood thinner than to do the greatest good for the most people.

According to PhRMA, as previously mentioned, the high cost of new medications is justified by the high costs of research and development. Not discussed by PhRMA is the high cost of marketing, which now includes the burgeoning expense of direct-to-consumer advertising in the media. As long as the glow of scientific objectivity on the research used in the new drug application passes muster with the FDA, the opportunity is there to aggressively seek a share of the market for that class of drug. Of course, the mainstay of product marketing is directly to physicians, by drug sales reps visiting the office, by printed advertising in medical journals, by direct mail advertising, and by sponsorship of required continuing education courses that include a good dose of positive information about the new medication. Convincing the medical community to use a new medication depends upon a high-powered marketing approach, with sponsorship of meetings and dinner "roundtables with the experts" to introduce doctors to new advances.

Let us examine the sponsorship of continuing medical education programs for physicians by pharmaceutical companies. For example, a visiting medical professor is scheduled to speak at a noon education conference at a hospital auditorium. Doctors drift in to eat a buffet lunch and hear the latest discussion of "Outcome Analysis in the Treatment of Migraine Headache." The speaker may actually do clinical research on migraine. Or, the pharmaceutical company may recruit a noted neurologist who is a skilled speaker to give the lecture. In either case, the company provides a significant "honorarium" to the speaker. The data presented often include the advantages of the new and extremely expensive migraine drugs produced by the pharmaceutical company over older agents. The day's educational lesson seems to be that this company's new medicine is much more effective than that of any other company or of the older generic, less expensive medicines. What information would be presented if the "continuing education" session were presented by a researcher or speaker not supported by *any* pharmaceutical company? There is actually a large body of data demonstrating that over-the-counter medications containing acetaminophen and caffeine can shut off a migraine at least 75 percent of the time for pennies per dose, but the demand for the new, $15-per-dose boutique-style medications continues to grow.

Doctors are not the only ones under the direct or indirect influence of the pharmaceutical industry. Marketing strategies of the pharmaceutical companies include a heavy-hitting effort to ramp up their share of the action by inducing patients to ask their doctors for the new, expensive, exciting agents as first choice treatment. Once, federal law restricted advertising to consumers. With repeal of this regulation through PhRMA lobbying efforts, the door was opened for the blitz of direct-to-consumer campaigns. Advertising has had a significant effect on generating demand. The promise of a magic panacea of instant relief appears on the television screen. The patient is highly motivated to ask the doctor about trying out the new wonder for migraine she or he has seen on television: "Ask your doctor whether a trial of MigraineBopper is right for you!" Commercials dance around the point of telling the patient that the new medication is a "sure bet." And the doctor has had the drug MigraineBopper appear before him in printed advertising in medical journals, in brochures from the sales rep, and he or she has heard it touted at educational meetings as producing substantial relief in 20 minutes or less in 72 percent of migraine headache episodes. In recent years, the expansion of drug coverage as part of health insurance has contributed to the rise in demand for expensive, new medications. If the net cost of that $15-per-dose new migraine drug is reduced to $2 per dose because of a drug insurance plan, the patient has further incentive to try the medication, as there is almost "nothing to lose." The ordinary economic forces of supply and demand determining price have been completely detached from the decision to prescribe and ingest a very expensive migraine pill. Strangely, the pill may be no more effective than an over-the-counter mixture of pain drug and caffeine. We, as doctors and patients, have been manipulated into pursuing "the best outcomes money can buy" on behalf of an industry. The "Truth" with a capital "T" as to the best treatment with the best outcome for the lowest cost for the entire population continues to elude us.

Your Doctor Is a Nurse

When the GP of the 1950s seemed to walk on water, his patients thought that he knew "everything." Certainly, he had detailed knowledge of his long-term patients and could handle the majority of their health issues by himself. Many experienced doctors develop a sixth sense about illness, being able to rapidly diagnose the one patient in 10 with a life-threatening problem, while the other nine patients with the same symptom can be reassured that their illness is not serious. As medical care became more complicated in the 1960s and 1970s, there were still strong figures in the "primary care" specialties manning the front lines in offices, caring for volumes of patients each week, but relying more on consultations with subspecialists dealing exclusively with one body part. The term "general practitioner" was officially retired in 1969, to be replaced by "family practitioner." Other specialists assumed the primary care role for selected portions of the population.

For children, the pediatrician became the primary care doctor. Earlier, when pediatricians were fewer in number, they functioned as a consultant to the general practitioner in complicated cases. Gradually, the expanding three-year pediatric residency programs turned out more pediatricians, and pediatricians took over more and more of the primary care of children.

For adults, the primary care specialty is internal medicine. The term "internal medicine" is somewhat confusing. Perhaps "adult medicine" would be a better name for the specialty. "Internist" sounds like "intern." "Intern" is the now obsolete term for first year trainee just out of medical school, like Dr. Kildare, for those who remember the old television series. Internists also do a three-year training program called a residency before starting practice.

The old GPs had a one-year rotating internship after medical school. The newer specialty of family practice was established in 1969 in an attempt to train doctors to carry on the tradition of the GP in treating patients of all ages. There are currently three years of residency training after medical school, with exposure to all aspects of the care of children and adults. For a while, family practitioners were even doing deliveries, but those doctors in charge of the more technologically complicated "birth centers" have tended to keep obstetricians in control and to exclude the family practitioners.

Many people in the United States are still cared for and are loyal long-term patients of one of these primary care doctors, a pediatrician, internist, or family practitioner. But here in the San Francisco area, we are watching the primary care physicians disappear. How can this be happening? Falling incomes, rising expenses, the burden of regulatory paperwork, and the inverted incentives of managed care all take their toll on doctors. Residents completing their training no longer seek to enter a practice. Rather, they find a salaried niche in an academic program, a county or Veteran's health program, or a closed-panel HMO, and hunker down, waiting for better times. More and more patients are simply unable to hook up with a primary care doctor who is readily accessible and follows them over the long haul. Conversely, patients may be forced by the provisions of their insurance plan to get care from the family practitioner that might be better provided by a doctor with subspecialty training.

Managed care companies in the 1980s started to refer to medical care as a "product." The product had to be delivered at the cheapest unit price. The goal in health care became "cost-effective, efficient care," yet the outcome looks quite different to me, more like "cheaper, inaccessible, delayed care, given reluctantly at great cost when you finally are really sick." In the new vocabulary of cost control, doctors have become "providers," and as other personnel have been substituted for doctors, "health professional" has become another buzzword for the person providing care to the patient.

With the tremendous financial pressures on individual doctors, doctor groups, and hospitals, the 1990s saw an acceleration of cost-containment measures. Among these was a dilution of the level of training of the "health professional" at the bedside or examining table of the patient. Nurse practitioners and physician assistants were recruited to see patients instead of doctors. In the hospital, bedside duties formerly performed by a registered nurse (RN) were delegated to a "direct care technician," someone in a uniform with the most minimal training in how to use an automated blood pressure cuff and thermometer.

There is a certain irony in the evolution of these changes. I previously discussed how family practitioners were squeezed out of the delivery room by the obstetricians, who claimed that the technology had become more complicated and required a specialist specifically trained in the area. When the notion of using non-M.D.s as a substitute for the obstetrician first came up in the 1980s, I heard one veteran obstetrician comment "Over my dead body." But the fees allowed by the insurers for the management of labor and delivery steadily fell, and this same obstetrician welcomed the change in hospital bylaws that permitted a nurse-midwife (a licensed form of "health professional" in California) to attend uncomplicated vaginal deliveries without a doctor present. As of this writing, doctors still are required to perform Cesarean sections, but in the near future a specialized nurse-expert position will be created to do this procedure.

An increasing proportion of the population sees a nurse practitioner or physician assistant as their "primary health provider." A seasoned and concerned nurse practitioner is often indistinguishable in manner and performance from a doctor, both from the patient's perspective and as measured by the outcome of care provided. For routine problems, conforming to typical textbook diagnosis and treatment protocols, everything goes fine. I have noticed that when a situation gets complicated or unusual, however, the less experienced "provider" may not get a handle on the diagnosis and treatment of the case. People are not textbooks. There are diverse and subtle meanings to the symptoms and behaviors of patients that take many extra years of training and experience to understand. So it is the less typical patient, or the one with multiple chronic illnesses, who falls through the cracks. An opportunity to diagnose and treat a developing serious problem at an early phase is missed, and the patient becomes one more case transported horizontally to the overcrowded emergency room in a truck with red lights.

Some may accuse me of sexism in distinguishing the performance of a doctor and a nurse practitioner in a complicated patient, but I don't consider the sex of the "health care provider" to be at issue. Fifty years ago, most doctors were male and most nurses were female. There were stereotypes of professional performance and gender that distinguished one from the other quite clearly. Very few women were accepted into medical school through the 1950s, and I have heard firsthand reports of the discrimination and abuse that women in medicine were subjected to in that era. Likewise, there were very few men in nursing, and those who chose to go to nursing school were derided for their lack of masculinity. Luckily, we have moved somewhat closer to egalitarianism in health care over the years. I have had the privilege of working alongside numerous fine physicians who happened to be women and many fine nurses who happened to be men. So, for the sake of this discussion, any non-egalitarian hierarchies that I dwell upon have nothing to do with the sex of those concerned. I do perceive a difference in the degree of competency between the typical primary care M.D. and the typical nurse practitioner, even if each has spent an equal number of years in the workplace. The length and breadth of the training is considerably longer for the doctor than for the nurse, and the level of responsibility borne by the doctor is much higher. In fact, the doctor is always the individual with the ultimate responsibility for the outcome of the care of the patient, even if he delegates part of the patient's care to another professional.

Supposedly, nurse practitioners work under the supervision of a doctor at all times. In everyday reality, a busy doctor is seeing patients at a vigorous pace, and the nurse practitioner working with him is seeing patients autonomously. Everything the nurse practitioner does is over the doctor's signature, but the signature may be on blank pre-signed prescription blanks and laboratory requisition forms. It is the economics of health care that is driving the substitution of doctors with other personnel. A nurse practitioner may earn more than a nurse on a general medical floor in a hospital, but the income is lower than that of the doctor.

After 20 years of touting a huge excess of physician supply, the health policy experts are finally noticing that there is a doctor shortage. By 1980, various studies published by the experts warned that an excess of doctors was developing that would increase health expenditures and have a negative impact on the economy. One factor that they did not accurately foresee was the unexpected increase in the U.S. population, which reached 285 million people in 2000, exceeding projections by more than ten percent. This lowered the overall ratio of physicians per 1000 of the population to 2.7, a number considered marginally low. We have gone full circle. In the 1960s, there was a perceived doctor shortage, made more obvious to the general public and the policy makers by the disappearance of the friendly GP. After huge resources were allocated to producing more doctors, an excess of supply, doing too many expensive procedures on too many patients, was the worry of the 1980s. Medical school class sizes were shrunk. Residency positions were gradually eliminated. Now we are on the verge of a crash program to increase the number of M.D.s. Unfortunately, in my opinion, most of the new trainees will be encouraged to enter subspecialty training. The percentage of active physicians in a primary care role has fallen from 67 percent in 1970 to 50 percent in 2000, according to statistics from the American Medical Association.[1] We will likely rev up the supply of cardiologists, gastroenterologists, and plastic surgeons. Some of the policy makers actually believe this would be the proper outcome and that we should replace M.D.s in the primary care specialties like internal medicine, family practice, and pediatrics with "advanced-practice nurses." I have argued that nurse practitioners have less training and experience than M.D.s. While this is not an issue in 19 out of 20 patient encounters for routine illnesses, it is the twentieth patient, the one with the unusual or atypical dis-

---

1.   AMA (Data Resources) Physician Statistics. Available at http://www.ama-assn.org/ama/pub/categroy/2688.html

ease that has the better chance of early diagnosis and treatment with the services of an M.D.. Missing the opportunity for early intervention can be very costly, as measured in dollars and in less tangible emotional stress to the patient and family. Even if the illness is non-life threatening, a missed diagnosis in the office can mean an emergency room visit later at ten times the cost of an office visit.

The value of thorough primary care was noted by the physician Maimonides (1135-1204 AD). In *The Regimen of Health Care; 4:7-8* he states:

Any intelligent person can study medical literature and understand when or when not to use various treatments. What is so difficult, even for a skilled physician, is to apply this knowledge in individual cases. For those who know nothing about the fundamentals of healing and treat it casually and talk a lot, nothing seems difficult. They don't think there is any illness that requires careful deliberation...Medicine...is really extremely difficult to master even for a conscientious physician.

How true these words seem today, even as the health policy makers, sitting in their ivory tower isolation, plot how to cheapen health care with the use of personnel less trained than M.D.s to make decisions previously thought to require M.D.s.

Another irony in the substitution of nurses for doctors is the disappearance of much-needed nursing personnel from the inpatient hospital setting. The nursing shortage in 2002 has become acute in California and other areas of the U.S., with hospitals extremely short-staffed. Ever more nurses are doing the work of doctors such as administering anesthesia or delivering babies. An increasing percentage of nurses are employed full-time performing administrative duties, in preference to the stresses of the overcrowded hospital wards. Each RN on the floor has had to cope with a greater volume of patients, sicker patients, and ever increasing charting responsibilities. A common complaint from patients is that "No one ever came into my room when I was in the hospital." These days, it is common for the harried staff to be seen clustered around computer terminals, doing the required charting, more frequently than they are seen with the patient. Performance is judged by the timeliness of the computerized charting of medication administration and vital signs.

Where are the nurses? The general population is growing. People are living sicker, longer (or is that longer, sicker?), spending more days in some kind of health care facility. Nursing school output has not kept up with the increasing need. As nurses get more experience, they opt out of the high-stress hospital shift work in favor of nurse practitioner, public health, administrative and specialized outpatient positions. Within the hospital, more nurses are doing jobs formerly done by doctors, such as delivering babies, assisting at surgery, and administering anesthesia. In each case, the initial protest of the doctor groups concerned is over-come by the falling reimbursement rate for the procedure involved. If you lower the fee for anesthetizing a patient for surgery sufficiently, the doctors with a spe-cialty in anesthesiology become willing to relinquish their turf to the nurses, now retrained as "nurse-anesthetists." If the care of a patient population is capitated, that is, a fixed fee per patient per month is given to the anesthesiologists to per-form any and all anesthesia necessary, they rally to change the rules to substitute nurses for themselves. Money remains a powerful motivator of group behavior. Capitation poisons the motivation for peak performance in patient care by removing any direct reward for excellence in professional duties. The "dumbing down" of the entire system, driven by short-term financial concerns, is a major force in the decline of health care quality in the United States. Yes, we are all multi-potential beings. Michael Rosenblum M.D. is fairly handy with home plumbing and can bumble through changing an O ring on a faucet without flooding the house. As far as taking a propane torch and sweating twelve joints on copper pipe to connect a new hose bib, he prefers to call a master plumber. The person with training and experience does the job in one-tenth the time, and the new pipe does not leak. In the same way, substitution of lower-paid professionals for doctors works when the problem is simple. When the disease is complex, the most highly trained and experienced M.D. should be there at the front lines of care to sort out the problem.

In California, the doctors on the front lines are disappearing. A recent survey by the California Medical Association seems to suggest that a significant number of currently practicing physicians will retire, move out of state, or switch careers in the next few years.[2] The health policy makers will look upon this trend as another reason to substitute doctors with nurse practitioners and other health professionals, claiming that the performance of the other professionals is indistin-guishable from that of the M.D.s. I suspect that this notion will ultimately be proven false and that delay in treatment will generate huge costs for the occa-sional complicated patient who needs early and aggressive intervention. The cost of many days of intensive care treatment, delivered too late, will more than offset the short-term savings from the use of less expensive personnel. It is the astute primary care doctor who keeps all the diagnostic possibilities in mind when con-fronted with a patient with puzzling symptoms. It is the experienced doctor who can sort through the haze of twelve miscellaneous symptoms and realize that the anxious patient is actually having atypical signs of a pending heart attack. Making

---

2.   http://www.cmanet.org/upload/Physician_Supply_(Acrobat).pdf

a difficult diagnosis depends on having seen a broad spectrum of common and not-so-common diseases during medical school and training and bearing the responsibility for diagnosing and treating them. Many hours of patient care crammed into the days and nights allow the doctor to experience a patient with a particular unusual disease, or an unusual presentation of a common disease, once or twice in his or her career. The nurse practitioner simply has not had the opportunity to care for such a patient. The trend of the past 10 years, to cheapen care at the front lines, has been driven by short-sighted economic factors. Money from health insurance premiums that should go to patient care has ended up in the earnings column of the financial statements of health management companies. The patients are the ones who are neglected at the front lines of care. Now, they fill the emergency rooms and acute hospital beds.

Your Hospital Is a Health System

When a serious and frightening illness strikes us, we would like to think of a hospital as the place where we receive help and hope and care. Yet, the recent headlines seem to paint a different picture of hospitals.[1] Instead of providing care, producing profits has become the major concern.

Hospitals have gone through a major evolution over the past 100 years. At the start of the twentieth century, most medical care was administered in a doctor's office or at home. Many people were born at home and died there in their own bed. When the Flexner Report of 1910 standardized and improved medical education and training, much of the training of medical students and interns was done at large county hospitals affiliated with the revamped medical schools. These large, busy hospitals served mainly an indigent population of patients, who, while receiving care, became a captured audience for the benefit of new doctors-in-training. Many of these institutions still exist, and in medical circles, their names are legendary: Boston City Hospital, Bellevue Hospital (New York City), Philadelphia General Hospital, Cook County Hospital (Chicago), Charity Hospital (New Orleans), and San Francisco General Hospital are a few examples. When these hospitals were at their pinnacle, they each had thousands of inpatient beds in operation. To patients, they have always been bustling and formidable places. Typically, these institutions consisted of distinctive high-rise brick towers sprawled over many city blocks. I still get a sense of foreboding when I am in the vicinity of one of these General Hospital complexes, though many have been modernized and are smaller in size than the old brick towers.

When the county hospitals had their highest patient census, in the first half of the twentieth century, there was a friendlier "private" class of hospitals used by GPs to serve their paying customers. Many of these private facilities started as "cottage hospitals," handfuls of beds in rambling wooden houses, modified to include operating room and patient areas. For the minority of cases that could not be treated by the GP at home or in the office, the patient was sent to the cot-

---

1. Reed, A. Tenet hospital in California is searched by U.S. agents. *NY Times*, November 1, 2002.

tage hospital in rural areas or the small community hospital in urban areas. This type of small hospital, with dour nurses in starched white uniforms and white caps, was the place you were cared for after a heart attack or if you needed your gallbladder removed. It was where the general surgeon operated on patients referred by the GP. I remember knowing of general surgeons in the 1950s who did "everything" at community hospitals, not only treating appendicitis and inflamed gallbladders, but also handling major fractures and performing skin grafts on patients with third-degree burns. These days, there are separate surgical subspecialists, namely orthopedic and plastic surgeons, respectively, for fractures and burns. In retrospect, it was a kinder, gentler, and simpler world for the patient of the 1950s, and the overall cost per day was a tiny fraction of today's hospital charges. However, for many complicated illnesses there was very little that could be done for the patient. Indeed, many patients died at comparatively early ages from diseases that are now readily treatable with recent medical advances. New advances come with a high price sticker.

The medical landscape began to change after World War II. The population of the U.S. swelled. War refugees arrived in numbers. The great Baby Boom began. New suburbs sprang up around the old inner cities as the automobile became the major form of transportation. And the promise of new technology to cure disease excited the public. Most care was still given by GPs, but as television invaded the nation, the miracle of new heart surgeries to correct diseased valves could be viewed in one's living room. The idea of seeing a "specialist" for troubling symptoms became a desirable option for patients.

Federal dollars began to subsidize new hospitals in the suburbs. The perception of a shortage of doctors led to huge subsidies for medical education and training. The nation willingly pumped increasing money into the health care industry, with images of disease-free survival to age 100 instilled into the mass consciousness. The hospital became a magical place where "they" did amazing things to your body. If you broke your hip, no longer were you confined to bed-rest for six months with a 50 percent chance of dying during the ordeal. Now, a stainless steel hip prosthesis could be inserted surgically to replace the shattered hip and you would be upright within a week. And it was no longer old Dr. Spivey, the GP who knew everything, performing these acts of magic. Dr. Spivey was never trained to do complicated joint surgeries. It was a highly specialized, recently trained orthopedic surgeon who was called in to "do the case." Perhaps the surgeon was a little impersonal, but he knew how to perform elaborate surgical repair and replacement of joints. Dr. Spivey had available only plaster casts and splints for joint injuries. The orthopedic surgeon required the increasingly elaborate facilities of the modern hospital, with specialized equipment and specially trained staff. Likewise, in every specialty area of patient care, the capital cost of setting up part of a hospital to do the new procedures and the ongoing costs of personnel caused hospital budgets to skyrocket.

The community hospitals did well in the fee-for-service era of the 1950s, '60s, and early '70s. Room charges rose from $30 per day to $60 per day, to $200 per day for a standard two-bed room, and to $1000 per day for intensive care during these three decades. Insurance paid for a greater and greater percentage of the cost for a larger and larger percentage of the population. The hospital was the place to go if you were sick, and now a vast majority of the population was born there and died there. The phenomenon of birth and the inevitable last breaths of life were no longer part of everyday experience. These were sequestered away in sparkling new community hospitals with those nurses in starched uniforms and caps, and bad things happened, out of sight of the rest of society, in the rooms on either side of a hushed corridor with a polished floor. Not until a more voyeuristic shift in popular culture occurred would a new generation get to see blood and gore and fancy life support equipment displayed in detail on weekly real-life TV series.

The nation's economic troubles in the 1970s began to impact the community hospitals. The sudden rise in energy costs and energy-driven inflation squeezed operating margins. The number of patients needing life-saving care who were uninsured began to increase. The safety net of Medicaid only provided a fraction of the cost of care, as the fee schedule was frozen and then reduced by cash-strapped federal and state government structures that were not lobbied by recipients of Medicaid services. The new technologies introduced in the 1950s and 1960s were trickling down through the health care systems, from the university hospitals to larger, regional community hospitals, and then to smaller community hospitals. The capital required to start up programs like open-heart surgery or neonatal intensive care was significant, and suddenly, in the 1970s, capital was in short supply. Local philanthropy had always been a source of help to the smaller hospitals, but now it was inadequate for funding the buildings and equipment needed to stay up-to-date.

Profitable ancillary and outpatient services were introduced by community hospitals to supplement the sagging income from inpatient care. Physical Therapy and Diabetic Education are examples of services that could be ordered by an M.D. for an outpatient and administered at an outpatient facility operated by the hospital and staffed by non-M.D. health professionals. "Hospital" became an archaic term for the expanding array of services at the community hospital. Many were renamed "Medical Center" to connote the range of treatment available in addition to the care provided in inpatient beds.

From my vantage point, external destructive forces began to intrude into the previously sacred territory of the hospital by 1980. Insurance companies instituted contractual reductions in fees as the PPO plans created a captured audience of insured patients. Hospital administration felt obligated to sign the contracts, to be a "preferred hospital" for the insurance plans. Managed care companies initially demanded straight discounts from the standard fee-for-service items tallied on the bill of each patient. Then, with the inception of capitation, the managed care company provided the hospital with a fixed monthly payment per "covered life" per month. No longer could the hospital bill for itemized charges for each patient each day. Hospital administrators felt obligated to participate in these schemes or else lose "patient base." High-paid consultants recommended signing every capitated plan available, to reach a minimum threshold of "covered lives" required to provide "cost effective services of value to the community" and permit economic survival of the hospital. Administrators believed that to not sign meant financial destruction of the hospital. The increasing numbers of patients with managed care insurance had to go to their "designated health care facility", an institution that had signed a contract with the patient's insurance plan, or risk not being covered for a hospitalization.

Hospitals began to lose money on large segments of the patient population they served. By the early 1990s, some community hospitals were closing. Those not closing had to consider a new option, that of joining a "Health System." What is a Health System? It is often an investor-subsidized, for-profit, public corporation that runs hospitals and outpatient facilities. In theory, a large Health System could get higher payments from large insurance and managed care companies by being able to service a large pool of capitated patients in a geographical area. The care could be delivered at lower unit cost due to the alleged economies of scale in a large operation.

As I write this in 2002, many Health Systems remain fiscally stressed. The economies of scale have not been realized. Huge expenses for new data processing equipment, for compliance with ever-increasing regulations, and for the rising costs of a scarce nursing staff are threatening the economic survival of many Systems. To the communities served by hospitals now operating as units in a System, the financial stresses may not be apparent. Glossy brochures are mailed to each household touting the high-tech yet personal and friendly service of the Health System, urging patients to designate it as the preferred institution in their health plan. Some Health Systems operate component community hospitals on a not-for-profit basis and solicit contributions on behalf of the local unit. But to those with knowledge of patient care operations inside the buildings, the decline in quality is apparent.[2]

The economic realities of the present create delay and inconvenience for patients needing specialized care. Certain money-losing services are closed at particular facilities within the Health System. One may have to drive an extra 20 miles to get the outpatient scope surgery on one's knee or even to give birth. This decrease in convenience and accessibility is termed "consolidation of services." The loss of such facilities as a Birth Center in one community hospital unit of a multi-hospital system is touted as providing "a higher level of specialized intensive care services" at the more distant facility to which patients now must go. A registered nurse-specialist often carries out services that used to be performed by a doctor. A significant portion of inpatient care is given by technicians and aides rather than registered nurses. A new industry of "Quality Assurance" has sprung up to document the outcome of care and to follow up on mistakes in care. Outside agencies, some governmental and some independent, require this information to "accredit" the Health System and allow its continued operation. Some unknown yet significant proportion of health care dollars disappears into the black hole of compliance and quality assurance. With the press full of reports of errors in hospital care causing sickness and death[3], there is public clamor for even more record keeping and reporting, as though this would provide more nurses at the bedside.

Clearly, the entire story of the Health System has not yet been played out. Larger, more impersonal institutions seem to be evolving, despite the glossy brochures marketing personal service. The rise in harmful mistakes made on hospitalized patients grabs the headlines. Personally, I am not convinced that there are economies of scale above a certain size of hospital. That size may be an autonomous community hospital of 450 beds. The promised savings from multiple institutions of this size combining into a "System" have not been realized. New layers of administration are required to run a group of hospitals, separated by miles from each other. A lot of unnecessary effort and expense is put into standardizing décor, procedures, and paperwork at each member institution. Sometimes, the housing of this entire administrative infrastructure requires a massive office building separate from all the hospital buildings. My personal desire is to

2.   Cohn, J. Sick: Why America is losing its best hospitals. New Republic May 28, 2001, pp20-25.

3.   Leape LL. Institute of Medicine medical error figures are not exaggerated. *JAMA.* 2000;284:95-97.

end this rush to "bigger is better," and return to a cycle of friendlier, moderate-sized community hospitals that operate with more patient care and less overhead.

However, there is the continuing problem of raising capital. Only larger Health Systems have access to the investor capital that appears to be essential for building and maintaining facilities, purchasing expensive high-tech equipment, and establishing the complex infrastructure, like information technology systems, needed to operate a patient-care institution in the present day. Where does this money come from? The answer, increasingly, is Wall Street. Issuance of stock by health management companies who own hospital systems funds a larger and larger fraction of the capital costs of hospitals. Is this desirable? It may be the only way to continue to have adequate facilities for inpatient care. It does raise the question of for whom the hospitals now exist. Should they be a profit center for shareholders of a corporation headquartered a thousand miles away? There are arguments for and against the current trend of using private capital. I have already stated my bias toward local control and funding, but I may have an unrealistic expectation of the adequacy of local funding.

Occupancy rates in community hospitals have risen dramatically in the last several years. By 1997, many community hospitals had occupancy rates under 60 percent. The trend toward lower occupancy frightened many institutions into becoming part of larger Health Systems. Then, the trend to greater numbers of emergency room visits, more admissions, and higher occupancy rates began. One can debate the causes of the sudden rise in bed occupancy. The unexpected increase in the U.S. population, fueled by immigration to supply manpower for the great "dot com" boom of the 1990s certainly played a role. But a major contributing factor was the switch of health care insurance to capitation in the 1990s. The "miracle" of managed care was supposed to provide quality health care at lower cost. Instead, it created incentives to minimize care, postpone care, do less thorough preventive care, and in general not diagnose and treat problems at an early stage. There were initial savings, with a major portion of the money going to the earnings of managed care companies. Then, the postponement of diagnosis and treatment began to bear a bitter harvest of patients with advanced disease showing up in the emergency room, needing admission to the hospital, and requiring the belated attention of many medical specialists. Since the Hospital System had already been paid for the care of the patient with a monthly capitation payment, the more expensive care now required put financial stress on the system. As I write this, a small revolt is in progress, with Health Systems attempting to drop capitated plans or have reimbursement switched to a per diem formula. There is somewhat of a trend away from capitated reimbursement to hospitals in favor of a discounted per diem rate. In other words, some insurance companies and hospitals would rather cope with the itemized bills for days of service than with the flat rate reimbursement under capitation. How this will play out over the next 10 years remains to be seen.

The shift to HMO-type insurance may have driven the formation of large hospital systems in the 1990s, but the current dependence on outside financing for such programs as the upgrading of buildings and the introduction of specialized services such as gamma knife radiation facilities and robotic operating facilities is likely to continue. Only large institutions, with many local hospital units, can raise the capital to afford these new technologies. The lure of surgery performed by a "robot" using "advanced laser technology" is advertised to consumers, who hope that the magic machines will provide a fast and successful surgery. The reality that it is a hands-on, labor intensive effort that determines successful outcome is lost. The headlines reporting deaths due to errors in the hospital are somehow detached from the supposed infallibility of the robot surgeon. Human hands, subject to error, are manipulating the robotic hands.

The friendly local hospital, ready and waiting should you need care, is becoming a memory, along with adequate nursing staff and personal attention.

The Collapse of Academic Medicine

Another story that is still being written is the ongoing destruction of medical schools and their affiliated teaching hospitals. When I entered medical school in 1969, a period of tremendous federal subsidization of medical education and training was underway. Health planners and economists had declared there to be a shortage of doctors, especially in rural and inner city areas. New medical schools were under construction, the class sizes of existing schools were being increased, and money was flowing into new specialty training programs to promote the new technologies. By 1979, economists feared a looming doctor excess rather than a shortage, and the flow of money into the medical schools began to slow.

The academic realm is a strange world of hierarchical power. By this I mean that there are many rungs to climb on the ladder to success in a teaching institution. Success would be attainment of full Professor status in a clinical department, Chair of a department, or a position as Dean. Paradoxically, it is not excellence in the care of patients that qualifies one for these positions, nor is it excellence in teaching. The single most important standard in moving from Clinical Assistant Professor, to Associate Professor, to Professor, to Department Chair is the number of original research papers published. "Publish or perish" remains the credo of the career medical school faculty member. Obtaining grants to fund research, either from public or private institutions that issue them, has produced an ongoing epidemic of "grant anxiety" in the academic realm.

At the lowest rung of the ladder for full time faculty is the newly appointed Clinical Assistant Professor. At the lower end of the salary scale, this individual must see patients a number of hours a week in specialty clinics, along with the students and residents, and has other teaching duties peppered throughout his or her schedule. But the most important task is to find research grants and spend extra hours in the lab or at the computer in order to publish original studies. With gradual promotion to higher faculty positions, the burden of patient care and teaching is reduced and more time can be spent in the lab. Publication of important original research in a major journal not only leads to promotion at the medical school, but it also makes the acquisition of further grant money from government agencies, private charities, or pharmaceutical companies much easier.

One might say that there is a tradition of hazing in medical education and training that goes along with the steep vertical hierarchy in academic medicine. The lowest form of life in the professional realm in the teaching hospital is the medical student, always the source of free labor for menial tasks, and an easy target for humiliation by residents and faculty. How many hours did I spend holding retractors in a big operation during my surgery rotation in the third year of medical school? Once, when a case was not going well, the surgeon sent an instrument whizzing past my ear to bounce off the tiled wall behind me. How many faculty members glanced at fellow students and me with a contemptuous frown while pumping the chief resident for answers to obscure questions? The chief resident, in turn, has the privilege of demanding answers from the junior residents during less formal rounds.

Once one attains a faculty appointment, all the extra teaching duties at hospital rounds and conferences fall to the most junior faculty person. I have seen these people running around the wards, clinics, and conference rooms all day, and using the nighttime hours to catch up on their research and publishing.

The rigid system I have described works satisfactorily during times of generous funding. I have mentioned the flush of federal money that flowed through the university medical centers in the 1960s. By the 1980s, the flow had diminished considerably. By the 1990s, many major university medical center teaching hospital complexes were losing huge amounts of money per year. For those medical schools that are state-funded, the state government was underwriting the losses. In the economic boom of the '90s, the states were able to make up for operating losses in many cases. Now, with a slower economy and declining tax revenues in 2002, programs are being trimmed in an effort to cut budget deficits.

In California, we witnessed the preposterous merger of two medical schools in the San Francisco area in an ill-fated effort to stem a tide of red ink in each institution. The University of California-San Francisco School of Medicine, a state-funded institution, merged with Stanford University School of Medicine, a private institution 30 miles to the south of San Francisco. Millions of dollars were spent on consultants and attorneys, and faculty at meetings planning the merger of the two institutions spent thousands and thousands of hours of time trying to meld the two very different institutions. Supposedly, clinical services would be combined and duplicate facilities eliminated to produce huge savings in the operating budget. I have spoken with several faculty members from both institutions who were frustrated by the endless travels back and forth between the two campuses through heavy traffic, with meetings going on well into the evening.

The merger was dissolved after a couple of years. The total cost of the failed merger was in the hundreds of millions of dollars. The UCSF School of Medicine had to close a major affiliated community teaching hospital as a result, and Stanford University School of Medicine has eliminated some programs and is reducing many others.

It has been a long decline since the magical days of the 1950s and 1960s, when the new medical technologies of that era received the same attention as a walk on the moon. My wife recalls her cousin undergoing open-heart surgery in 1958 at a major university teaching hospital to repair a congenital heart defect. For the patient and her family, it was a spectacular and frightful ordeal, as though the patient were taking a dangerous walk in outer space. The heart surgeon was a super god at the pristine new hospital with its brand new intensive care unit, in which the patient remained for two weeks after the surgery. Cards and letters poured in from far and wide as total strangers heard of the major event and wanted to wish the patient a speedy recovery. The improvement in prognosis for the cousin was dramatic after the successful surgery, with the prospect of a full and symptom-free life, rather than shortness of breath and an early death.

Those early years of new technology made the university hospitals the "tertiary referral centers" for all the difficult cases that could not be helped at the local community hospital. The GP caring for the patient had already consulted a cardiologist at a secondary institution, who deemed it necessary to proceed with referral to the tertiary source of care. With the rise of indemnity health insurance in that era, for most patients with a serious condition "insurance would take care of everything."

Many medical schools developed a dual and two-class patient population. The big county hospitals with which they were affiliated were the main source of teaching and training patients, most of whom did not have any private insurance. These were the ancient crumbling brick buildings with the 30-bed wards. The indigent people in the adult wards had cirrhosis of the liver and infections from bad injection needles, and the pediatric wards had cases of meningitis, asthma, and lead poisoning. The new sparkling University Hospital nearby had two-bed hospital rooms with TVs, and the patients had less common problems like heart defects and rare tumors requiring the most expert specialized care. Medical students, interns, and residents had the opportunity to rotate through these different environments during their training.

With the inception of Medicaid in 1967, reimbursements to the university hospital for the care of the indigent improved and helped fund the expansion of training programs. However, with the economic woes of the U.S. through the 1970s, the indigent population without private insurance grew and fees under Medicaid were frozen and scaled back. Patients on Medicaid who could no longer receive care in their local communities for rather common illnesses would travel considerable distances to the university medical center affiliated county hospitals, where no one was refused care. Eventually, the fiscal deficits generated by providing care to the uninsured and underinsured put many county hospitals in jeopardy. The "social safety net" of the county teaching hospital developed many holes.

The generous subsidies for medical education enjoyed by students in the 1960s and early 1970s have long since disappeared. Medical school tuition exceeds $30,000 per year in many institutions. Tuition and living expenses for many students are financed by student loans. Many students graduate from medical school these days with student loan debt in excess of $100,000. With falling incomes among practicing physicians, default by borrowers is becoming more common. The phenomenon of financially strapped physicians declaring bankruptcy is no longer restricted to established M.D.s making stupid investment mistakes, a time-honored professional hazard. It is the newer generation of doctors who may never be able to provide themselves and their families with a comfortable and debt-free living.

Medical schools are reducing the number of students in each class and shrinking certain residency and postdoctoral programs. In one of the long cycles of the last half-century, we have gone from the perception of an extreme doctor shortage in the United States to one of an excess. Yet, there is a critical nursing shortage now in 2002[1], and often nurses are trained in the same teaching institutions as doctors. It is now the nursing students who are getting the kinds of subsidies that I enjoyed during my medical education. The pendulum is starting to swing in the opposite direction for doctors as well, with the economists and health planners starting to notice a developing shortage of doctors once again. It is predictable that life will improve for medical students, as increased subsidies for medical education are once again made available. However, in the United States we tend to make changes only in the setting of a crisis. We will not see a full resurrection

---

1.   Berliner, HS, Ginzberg, E. Why this hospital nursing shortage is different. *JAMA* 2002;288: 2742-44.

of medical school status and funding until the shortage of doctors has become extreme and is hyped in the popular media.

My hope is for an increase in funding for primary care training of doctors when the future shift of public sentiment occurs. By preferentially funding residencies in family practice, internal medicine, and pediatrics instead of the high-tech subspecialties, it would be possible to rebalance the health care delivery system, emphasize prevention rather than treatment of disease, and put the health care dollar where it actually provides a return. Putting aside monetary considerations, treating people aggressively and early can prevent heart disease, or delay its onset, and can detect cancer when it is more easily treated. Reducing the prevalence of these common diseases requires improvement in patient lifestyles. A powerful impetus for change is the strong primary doctor figure. A primary care doctor can achieve smoking cessation in 50 percent of patients with consistent follow-up. Something about the long hours spent in the hospital with the victims of tobacco-induced illness inspires zeal in helping smokers quit. Smoking is probably the most reversible factor contributing to preventable disease, and a noticeable percentage of all health care dollars spent goes toward treatment of the health consequences of cigarette smoking.

But the every day challenge of helping patients quit smoking is not the area receiving the research grants and the focus of attention at the academic medical centers. Recent years have seen the field of human genetics move into the forefront in funding and interest. Once again, the promise of a new and expensive technology to provide *the answer* to human suffering has had the attention of the researchers and the media. The reasoning goes something like "As soon as we unlock the secrets of the humane genome, we will finally have an understanding of why people get cancer, Alzheimer's disease, and coronary disease, with the promise of new cures to follow." Of course, *the answer* is always more complicated than hoped. The gene sequences have been mapped, but now we need to study the locking and unlocking proteins that regulate gene expression to get the ultimate solution to disease. These areas of research have noble and expensive goals. I am impressed that it takes ever-larger sums of money to make ever-smaller increments of progress in staving off disease and death.

In the meantime, ordinary, treatable, routine problems in ordinary people do not get enough attention. It is much cheaper to get smokers to stop than it is to unravel the human genome. Achieving smoking cessation in half the current adult cigarette smokers might just save more money in the next 10 years than all the research into the human genome. The unglamorous task of counseling smokers gets little time or money in academic institutions. It is not the source of a lot of research grant money. Perhaps we have lost the focus at the medical schools regarding what is important in disease prevention.

The initial spectacular, headline-making new surgeries of the 1950s and 1960s have become everyday, almost assembly-line events. A patient undergoing open-heart surgery may spend 90 minutes in the operating room instead of eight hours. Time in the intensive care unit postoperatively, when all goes well, can be less than 12 hours. Patients get discharged from the hospital as early as the fourth day after open-heart surgery. If one adjusts for inflation, the fees paid by Medicare and private insurers for an open-heart procedure are a tiny fraction of what they were in 1960. We have all become accustomed to having such technology available, should we or our loved ones need it, and we assume it will be there just in case. We may no longer view it as special or spectacular. We may have come to resent the rising health insurance premiums that pay for these procedures (albeit at a deep discount) for those of us who do need them. Between caring for the medically indigent and caring for the patients with difficult problems at a deep discount, the medical schools and university-affiliated hospitals have been brought to the brink of annihilation.

I hope that some balance can be restored between the need for extreme specialization and the need for excellence in primary and preventative care in communities. I keep coming back to the point that good primary care is the backbone of a health care system. Training doctors to fulfill this role with excellence begins at the medical schools and their affiliated hospitals. Excellence in primary care of patients and in training others to do primary care tends not to be rewarded in the overspecialized, "publish or perish" hierarchy of the teaching institutions. Long-term reduction in health care costs and improvement in patient outcomes can only be achieved with the redirection of resources to excellence in primary care. The original goal of the reforms outlined in the Flexner Report had as a central theme the production of well-trained doctors who could do most things for most patients. Training in a specialized area would follow the basic education for those who wished to pursue it. We have lost this ideal in academic medicine. Much very specialized care at university medical centers is delivered by clinicians who "can't see the forest for the trees." They lack grounding in the total care of the patient, who now is dehumanized to "a fascinating case of horrendenoma" (a gallows humor neologism defined as "horrendous incurable tumor"). Aggressive treatment, geared to total assault on the largely fatal disease, brings visions of research grants to investigate the latest anti-horrendenoma drugs and a long list of publications about improving survival by two months in the unfortunate people with the condition. For all the money spent on horrendenoma treatment, vast numbers of patients could be provided with (boring) routine and preventative care, possibly preventing the development of horrendenoma later in some of them. To restore academic medicine, we need to restore the balance between treating the routine and mundane, and treating the difficult and obscure disease.

Where Have All the Doctors Gone?

Once upon a time, there was a tradition in the medical profession that the doctor worked until he died with his boots on. This was certainly the ethic of the general practitioners of my childhood, those giants who walked on water.

I have described some of the negative forces that are slowly grinding the profession into dust, reducing doctors to angry, paper-shuffling automatons, rewarded for a high volume of mediocre work and punished for exemplary care of the patient. Fundamental to the decline of the medical profession has been the transition to capitated health plans. As I have discussed, in the past 50 years there has been a profound change in the way health services are paid for. In the mid-twentieth century, a majority of medical services took place in an office or at home and were paid for with cash. The rise of indemnity insurance as an employer-provided fringe benefit changed health services to an entitlement, something mostly free, paid for by someone else. Seeing the doctor became a right, not a privilege. The insurance company was uninvolved in the patient's care. It provided *carte blanche* coverage of whatever the good doctor deemed medically necessary. Then, by the 1980s, the PPO or preferred provider organization was introduced. Doctors had to sign a contract to provide their services at a discount or risk losing patients to other doctors if they did not sign. The final phase of the change was the widespread introduction of health maintenance organizations, or HMOs, in which the roles of insurance company, patient, and doctor were changed dramatically. The insurance company no longer indemnified, or accepted risk, for the payment for illness. It became a "health management company." It managed money, not health. The patient was no longer an insured human being, but became a "capitated life." The doctor was no longer a caring professional, but a "provider," paid a low fixed monthly fee per capitated life.

As a caring professional, the doctor wants to do what is best for the patient. As a provider of service for capitated lives, the doctor needs to hide from the patients, service them as little as possible, delay or minimize diagnosis and treatment, and convince himself or herself that these actions are for "the common good." To encourage adoption of this new role, the health management companies provide a variety of roadblocks to providing payment for services for sick patients. Rationing through paperwork is an everyday reality for doctors.

So many of my colleagues have looked at the overall situation and have made plans for an early retirement or a career change. Some end up working for pharmaceutical companies. Others perform utilization review for insurance companies. Once-proud primary care doctors often end up in a "cash and carry" practice on the edge of mainstream health care: one example is treating obesity in a clinic that provides amphetamine-like drugs monthly to the overweight hordes. Another is operating an "Appearance Enhancement Center," devoted to treating wrinkles, age spots, spider veins, and other unwanted accessories of the fiftyish yuppie set. "Credit cards are gladly accepted. The nurse-specialist can see you now and remove all unwanted hair from the bikini line with the magic laser." Still another way for a doctor to pay the mortgage is to operate a "Pain Treatment Center," dealing with patients who have chronic pain and writing the elaborate controlled-substance prescription for just enough narcotic medication to get to another appointment next month. And then, there is the "alternative medicine practice," in which the doctor retails boutique vitamins from the office. Some M.D.s have enrolled in law school and passed the bar. These doctor-lawyers are highly sought after in areas like medical malpractice case evaluation and defense.

Recently, radiologists have been advertising "whole-body CT scans" to the public as a high-tech screening tool for finding disease at an early phase. Patients express a great interest in the scan, even though it is not covered by insurance, and can cost many hundreds of dollars. The promise of a magic computer-driven technology, outside the mainstream of medical care, easily accessible for a price, seems to attract attention. Whether a whole-body CT scan is actually useful as a screening tool for the general population is highly debatable. Arguably, a doctor who knows the patient would obtain a much better result by performing a careful medical history and exam each year. Specific tests, possibly including CT scans, might be ordered for specific problems that turn up on the exam. However, patients will continue to flock to diagnostic and treatment regimes that are not in the mainstream of health care, especially if the mainstream is difficult to access, unfriendly, and does not provide any ongoing contact between the primary doctor and the individual.

Some doctors have found a haven in regions of the U.S. friendlier than the population centers of the east and west coasts. While there is no data to verify the situation, it appears that care is more accessible for patients in states like Arkansas, Kentucky, and Tennessee, where the percentage of the population covered by

HMO plans is very low, and the doctor's overhead is much lower than in urban centers. Malpractice insurance problems vary from state to state. For example, liability problems are difficult in Florida, which also happens to have a high percentage of HMO patients in south Florida urban areas, so south Florida has become a very difficult place in which to practice.

One interesting phenomenon is the change in outlook when a doctor works for an insurance company or government agency regulating the actions of other doctors. It is human nature to take on the coloration or expectation of the role one is in. If you are in a bureaucracy, you think like a bureaucrat. We read in the press of a decline in corporate ethics and honesty in accounting practices. In recent years, the bottom line results have become the focus of many organizations. One cannot depend upon the goodwill of individuals to overcome a structure's lack of integrity.

I have observed rather marked changes in behavior in colleagues who have moved into salaried positions even part-time within a Health System or large doctor group. As clinicians caring for patients, these individuals were often exemplary in their concern, availability, and knowledge. They tended to be outgoing and affable. Suddenly, in a salaried position within the Health System corporation, they are in a position of power over their peers, performing administrative duties such as clinical outcome and utilization review. They are paid to berate colleagues who order too many consultations or procedures. They are privy to the problems of cash flow through the medical group. They seem aloof. Their vocabulary changes. No longer does the doctor take care of the patient. Now there are a Group and a System providing "services of maximum value," and "utilizing scarce resources wisely in a cost-effective manner." The jargon of the health policy makers and the economists has replaced discussion of a difficult case of pancreatitis. The overriding concern for money rather than health becomes the focus of the M.D..

"The beatings shall continue until morale improves" might be a good description of the circumstances under which the doctors in large medical groups work. Another sarcastic expression of the current medical scene under capitation is "No good deed shall go unpunished." Those doctors who can get out of practice are getting out. Those who feel that there is no choice but to carry on, regardless of the frustrations, are a sorry lot these days; they are angry, depressed, and tired as they extend the workweek to compensate for falling fees. They fantasize about the time when they, too, will be able to leave practice. Sometimes they tell me, "But it is still wonderful to help people," or "When I am in the exam room, it's just me and the patient, and nothing bothers me." Such is the glimmer of remaining professionalism.

According to the American Medical Association, there are more than 800,000 M.D.s in the United States, or about one M.D. per 350 people in the population. A busy primary care doctor can care for 1500 patients. At first glance, the nation seems well supplied with medical manpower. Yet, only a minority of doctors remain on the front lines, ready to see patients for urgent reasons today. The majority of M.D.s are specialists in one part of the body or another, seeing patients only on referral and often only after a long wait of weeks or months. As M.D.s opt for administrative positions and reduce or eliminate patient care time, the number of M.D.s actually available declines further. M.D.s at University Medical Centers may devote only a small fraction of their week to patient care, with research activities in the lab taking up the majority of their hours. There are medical specialists who do not actually see living patients, such as pathologists, who examine tissues and administer laboratory facilities, and there are specialists like radiologists, whose passing contact with patients is in the context of an X-ray or angiogram procedure ordered by another doctor.

Doctors who have remained in primary care practice spend an ever-increasing proportion of their patient care time doing administrative chores. The number of pieces of paper to shuffle, or bytes of digital information to input has increased exponentially in recent years. Even well-meaning administrators in federal agencies who would like to reduce the number and size of the forms are hobbled by the rules. In the case of paperwork for Medicare patients, efforts by administrators to show that a form is unnecessary or counterproductive fall under the rules of the "Paperwork Reduction Act." There must be public announcement and public hearings about the proposed collection of data required to reduce the existing paperwork. And paperwork must be kept and filed about the public hearings. We have reached the ludicrous state of tying up huge resources in maintaining paperwork to monitor the paperwork that monitors physician performance. As the system breaks down and physicians leave practice, new agencies and organizations are created to collect and analyze data about the shortcomings of the health care system. There seems to be no one left to take care of the patient. In the popular media, we hear of terrible mistakes being made in hospitals, sometimes with lethal results. The answer of the federal government to concerns about this phenomenon is to create a new agency to collect data on errors in hospitals, with new forms to fill out each time a mistake happens.

As discussed in the chapter "Your Doctor Is a Nurse," patients may not even see a doctor for routine outpatient care at an office. The health policy makers are promoting the idea of using substitutes like nurses, physician assistants, and physical therapists on the front lines. Doctors will be used as specialists and subspecialists, and no M.D. will function as the caring, available figure in the patient's care. Specialists will increasingly become technicians, performing procedures like coronary angiography and endoscopy, not really concerned about the overall course of the patient's life, but only about the body part covered by their expertise. As more medical students are shunted into years of subspecialty training, the fees for each of the specialized procedures that they are trained to perform will be reduced. Many of these procedures will then be farmed out to lower paid nurse-technicians. We will end up with an even more fragmented, impersonal system of health care delivery, with no one in charge of the patient's overall long-term health.

This unhappy scenario is already underway, and those doctors able to vote with their feet and move on to other career options are doing so. Meanwhile, the use of RNs in positions formerly held by doctors has enhanced an already critical nursing shortage. We have already reached a point at which the hourly compensation earned by a highly trained nurse-specialist exceeds that earned by some doctors. I expect that this trend will continue, to the point where young people will no longer see a career as a doctor as something prestigious or desirable.

Reversing the trend to fewer doctors requires restoration of the control of patient care and fees, and elimination of the senseless piles of paper on the front lines of primary care doctors. The argument that we would have rapidly rising health care costs if we deregulate is spurious; overall, I would expect significant savings from the diagnosis and treatment of disease at an earlier phase and the return of care to the efficient venue of the small doctor's office. The quantity of regulations must be reduced, however impossible this seems to an entrenched bureaucracy, the existence of which is justified by the need to create and monitor rules and regulations. Regulating the primary care doctors to extinction destroys timely access to health care. Small hundred-dollar illnesses then become $30,000 disasters needing a dangerous stay in the hospital for treatment.

The process of reducing paperwork is very difficult. It means that many government and health insurance employees will no longer have work to do. An example of the kind of mountainous paperwork that does not help patients and actually can hurt them is the variety of forms required for prescribing and dispensing narcotic painkillers. When old Doctor Spivey made house calls and injected the dying with morphine from his big black bag, he simply ordered the morphine from a pharmacist and paid for it. Now there is an empire of regulatory agencies, federal and state, to oversee the use of morphine and other narcotics with the goal of preventing these agents from being diverted to illegal street trade. There are special forms for the wholesaler, the pharmacist, and the doctor. The doctor needs to register with the federal Drug Enforcement Agency and pay for an annual license to prescribe narcotics. States have various licenses and special narcotic prescription forms. The new specialty of "pain control" exists basically because many doctors are unwilling to perform the paperwork required to keep patients with chronic pain supplied with medication. Pain control specialists develop an elaborate routine in the office to comply with the various federal and state regulations, and much of their practice involves visits by patients to get refills of special narcotic prescriptions.

It appears that legally manufactured narcotics still find their way to the street trade, but the most notable result of the regulation of prescribing practices has been that *patients in great pain often do not receive sufficient medication to relieve their misery*. The time, hassle, and possible regulatory violations induce doctors to prescribe non-narcotic, less potent agents when they should be prescribing narcotics.

Rather than reduce the paperwork, the answer of our government officials has been to create new agencies and new laws to mandate and monitor the treatment of pain. In California, it is now a legal offense if the doctor does not adequately treat pain. So, the doctor can be punished for not doing the piles of paperwork required to prescribe adequate narcotics and can be punished for not prescribing adequate pain medicine. Meanwhile, doctors and taxpayers are bearing huge costs related to the monitoring of narcotics for medical use. None of this effort helps sick patients today. Only if the taxpayers, who are all potential patients, demand the reduction or elimination of the myriad agencies clogging the system with paper will we begin to unravel the mess. Society has not come up with a method to control illegal drug use. Making legitimate use of painkillers seem like a criminal action is not alleviating the problem.

Solutions: A National Medical Database—Would One Truly Violate Your Privacy?

John Doe has been found unconscious in the street and brought into the emergency room by ambulance. You are the emergency room doctor on duty. Where do you begin? As in every common emergency situation, there are standard procedures for the diagnosis and treatment of the patient. In the case of an unconscious person, the task is particularly difficult because John Doe cannot provide a medical history and cannot answer questions.

The protocol in this case is to look for signs of the common medical causes of unconsciousness, such as stroke, disturbance of heart rhythm, insulin reaction, and alcohol or drug overdose. Vital signs are taken, blood is drawn, an IV (intravenous) line is started, and a careful examination of the patient along with laboratory results, electrocardiogram, and imaging studies such as a CT (computerized tomography) scan of the head will usually reveal the cause of the patient's problem. However, these procedures all take time, and some individuals brought to the emergency room don't have any to spare.

What if the patient arrived in the emergency room with his medical history encrypted in a magnetic strip on a medical ID card? Even simple information, such as a history of diabetes, would be very helpful in the common situation of the comatose patient.

When the Clinton administration suggested the use of a national medical ID card, the "smart card", a howl of protest arose from those organizations that champion privacy. The American Civil Liberties Union raised the specter of unknown snoopers having access to one's intimate health care data, information supposedly shared privately with a doctor and no other person.

Privacy has been an illusion since the rise of the era of health insurance in the 1950s. There has always been a "third party" looking into our personal medical issues, usually in an effort to limit the payment for medical services. The fine print in any health insurance contract includes a blanket release for the review of our medical records by representatives of the insurance company, who actually *do* peruse them without obtaining further explicit permission or even informing us. Copies of medical records are faxed day and night between doctors' offices and hospitals and insurance companies.

Doctors exchange information about patient problems constantly, in person, by phone, by fax, and to some extent by e-mail, and this often without the formal written consent of the person concerned. Implicit in the request for care is an individual's consent for her M.D. to discuss the case with specialists consulting on the matter. If it weren't, the M.D. could accomplish little for her. Such discussions are not always held discreetly. Hospital elevators are a notorious source of leaks of private information about critically ill patients in the hospital. I remember being chastised by one of my mentors for opening my mouth about an anonymous case of horrendenoma (a bad lethal cancer growing aggressively) while strangers were in an elevator with the two of us.

When Congress passed the Health Insurance Portability and Accountability Act in 1996 (HIPAA), it included legislation pertaining to the privacy of personal medical information and standards for the electronic transmission of medical information. Medical privacy protections were to be established by regulation after the solicitation of comments from interested parties, such as medical professional societies, insurance associations, hospital representatives, and attorney groups. The legislation was strongly backed by a number of organizations, including the American Civil Liberties Union (ACLU). The ACLU, in a statement issued February 28, 2001, stated that "medical records contain uniquely sensitive information about individuals, and the increasingly common storage of such records on computers poses a threat to medical privacy. In the absence of legal safeguards, the new technology allows for virtually unlimited access to medical records without patient consent. The ACLU believes that federal protections are needed to shield medical information from unauthorized disclosures."

The ACLU statement can be very appealing to those not immersed in providing health care. Each of us wants our intimate medical details seen only by those directly involved in our health care. There may be embarrassing or damaging details about our past that should not be accessible to outsiders.

However, the confidentiality of the doctor–patient relationship has been one of the basic professional ethical standards built in to medical practice. Now, a large Federal agency will define protections for medical information in the digital age. The HIPAA of 1996 gave the Department of Health and Human Services (HHS) the task of developing new and detailed standards for privacy in the absence of action by Congress by August, 1999. As Congress was unable to complete the job, it did in fact go to HHS. An overview of the results can be viewed online.[1] The thousands of pages of proposed standards can be viewed online as well, downloadable in segments due to the vast size. Whether any single individual will actually be able to read and understand the standards for privacy is highly debatable. But there will be federal employees enforcing them!

I expect that the obvious and hidden costs of compliance by doctors and hospitals will take a significant bite out of those dwindling health care dollars discussed previously in this book. I have seen a relatively small hospital hire a full-time attorney to deal with HIPAA regulations. Each time our employer or we pay insurance premiums for health care, concealed in the payments are regulatory and legal costs. What do we get for these dollars? Let us assume that one in a million patient encounters results in a potential breach of confidentiality, that is, the wrong person obtains private and potentially embarrassing data. Maybe someone standing around in line in a pharmacy hears that a neighbor he knows is getting a prescription for an antidepressant medication. Or, maybe a printed lab result showing an HIV-positive result for a well-known celebrity gets viewed by an unauthorized person who calls a member of the press. These can be devastating breaches of confidentiality. Can we ever give 100 percent assurance that they will be prevented? Is there a sum of billions of dollars that will absolutely eliminate the problem? Will the proposed regulations effectively prevent these sorts of betrayals? Probably not.

How much money *should* the United States spend to improve the situation? It appears that billions of dollars will be spent complying with and enforcing the HIPAA privacy regulations. I suspect that the cost of each significant breach prevented will be in the millions of dollars. Tens of thousands of new forms will be filled out each day to comply with the regulations. There may be a slight reduction in the leakage of private health care data, but there definitely will be a large increase in the bureaucracy and paperwork associated with basic doctor–specialist communications. Staff time in doctors' offices and hospitals will be diverted to filling in confidentiality forms and acquiring patient signatures. Staff time costs money and makes for long lines for patients.

The simple act of a doctor ordering blood tests will now require new forms for the patient to sign to grant the doctor the revocable privilege of viewing his or her confidential laboratory results. How many pieces of paper will we need to accomplish a simple test on blood cholesterol? Will we drown in a sea of paper, even as we attempt to comply with the "Paperwork Reduction Notice" stamped on the

---

1.   http://hhs.gov/news/press/2002pres/privacy.html

latest federally mandated forms? Isn't it ironic that we create new forms while digital technology is supposedly eliminating the need for paper? Well, perhaps the forms will be on a handheld screen, but a stored electronic record of all the forms will be required, thickening all of our electronic patient files sufficiently to require expansions and upgrades to all hospital and office systems and, inevitably, more computer support personnel. And what if "the computers are down" or "I'm sorry, Ma'am, it's not in the computer"?

My hope is that some mass intelligence will emerge on the subject of health care privacy and repeal vast portions of HIPAA related to privacy. Unfortunately, a whole new industry of "health care compliance" has been created. People who market themselves as experts in health care compliance lobby to keep ever more regulations coming, since each additional regulation gives them another opportunity to bill for the set-up of further paperwork.

A significant difficulty with the new privacy regulations is their interference with the development of a national medical database. They are directly counter to such a database and likely prevent its creation. We need to have health care data on all citizens in a central electronic storage location networked to a terminal at each and every site where patients are seen. Countless times I have cared for a seriously ill person who was unable to give a medical history. If only I had had access to old records instantly at a terminal! Or, if there were a medical smart card with the patient, the key facts, such as past conditions, medications, allergies, and recent lab data, would be available. Theoretically, "firewalls" can be created to both comply with the regulations *and* allow doctors to retrieve centrally stored data rapidly on everyone in critical situations. However, we now have thousands of pages of privacy regulations making proposals for a national medical database more difficult and more expensive.

A significant fraction of the health care dollar goes toward duplicated services because we do not have easy access to previous test results, office records, and medication lists when the patient is in an accident or has a sudden and expensive crisis. The trend away from the 24-hour availability of the primary physician who knows the patient is making the situation worse. The "smart card" is a viable option, but centrally stored data could be more extensive, complete, and available even in the absence of such a card.

In addition to its tremendous help during medical emergencies, a national medical database would allow the simplified collection of data to determine whether new medications or technologies are indeed having the presumed beneficial effect on the public. Assuming that medical history and exam findings, medication lists, and lab and X-ray results are entered in a universal format, data on the results of particular tests and treatments could be extracted from the database. The statisticians collecting the data would not need to know the identities of any of the patients involved in their data collection. We might actually be able to find out, for example, whether cholesterol-lowering drug "LowChol" reduces heart attacks and at what rate and whether it has hidden long-term side effects. Currently, pharmaceutical companies must fund separate research projects to collect these kinds of data in a statistically significant population of patients for each new medicine. The cost of this research is part of the high cost of drugs. With a national medical database, the costs of collecting information for a large sample of patients would be much less, and the results could be synthesized by independent instead of profit-driven reviewers. As previously mentioned, the collection and evaluation of statistically valid data ("outcome analysis") is used for the development of better treatment protocols ("evidence-based medicine"). Making truly cost-effective health care treatment decisions based on the medical experiences of the entire nation could potentially improve the health of the average person at tremendous savings over the years. Some currently accepted expensive treatments would be shown to be duds. Other simple, less expensive and less toxic treatments would be shown to have tremendous value. But we need the data, a lot of it, cheap, without the bias of the interested parties funding its collection, to validly analyze outcomes.

The ACLU, in its position paper of March, 2001,[2] stated "To be sure, most patients will readily authorize disclosure of their records for treatment and payment, but some patients may want to place conditions on the use of especially sensitive information for non-essential purposes…" A requirement that "doctors seek authorization provides an opportunity for patients to consider these important questions and, if necessary, negotiate the terms under which records may be disclosed."

This position is ludicrous. A doctor may have thousands of pieces of data on a patient. A simple set of blood tests on an adult (complete blood count, chemistry panel, and urinalysis) produces a printout of 40 lines of data. How many hours should the doctor spend with the patient deciding which results may be disclosed? Maybe the slightly high blood sugar reading shouldn't be disclosed to the insurance company, lest the patient be rejected for having a tendency to diabetes. But perhaps that is an issue more of health insurance reform than of patient privacy. Or, do you want your cancer treatment options delayed while you are pre-

---

2. The latest position papers of the ACLU can be viewed at http://www.aclu.org/, following the links under "Privacy and Technology" to "Medical Privacy".

occupied faxing forms and signatures back and forth to the office assistants of a specialist across the country, who by the time this is done has left for a conference, when originally she was available to speak with your physician immediately over the phone? How obsessive can we be over patient records? We can spend the entire health care budget on this type of issue, even though 99.999 percent of the time it really makes no difference at all. In addition, access to a national database by independent researchers depends on not having barriers at the point of care to obstruct the storage of data. Surely, we have taken the privacy issue to extremes, and as a society we had better rethink the issues.

Meanwhile, the story of John Doe had a happy ending. His real name was Herman Newman, and he had accidentally taken a double dose of his diabetes medication. As his blood sugar fell to a low level, he decided in his confusion to take a walk and this 60-year-old collapsed about three blocks from home. He was found a short time later by passersby, lying face-down, unconscious. The panel of emergency blood tests included a blood glucose determination. His blood glucose was only 32 in the emergency room, low enough to cause unconsciousness, but rapid correction to a normal value of 100 allowed him to recover rapidly and return home three hours later.

Solutions: A Database for Patients

A huge amount of medical information is now found on the Internet. I have seen doctors dismiss as worthless the handful of printed material offered by a patient after the patient and knowledgeable family had spent hours finding and downloading some very pertinent material about a difficult illness. "I know more than what is on the Internet. I'm a doctor." More enlightened doctors have taken the time to sort through the material and pick out the useful information, which may have included very useful suggestions for diagnosis and treatment.

In 2000, presidential candidate Al Gore was correct in lauding the virtues of the Internet as "The Information Superhighway." The quantity of useful information for patients and doctors is truly astounding and increasing all the time. I have found the information at the web site of the National Institutes of Health[1] particularly valuable. While the site is a bit difficult to navigate, one can find the latest reports on treatments for patients and doctors on major classes of diseases at each of the component institutes.

I have always thought that patients should be empowered with as much information as they can handle about their disease and its treatment. A good example of success with this style of care is in the treatment of diabetes. With self-monitoring of blood glucose using a small portable meter and test strips, much better control of the disease has been achieved by millions of patients, with improved outcomes for the prevention or delay of complications.

We have entered the age of direct-to-consumer advertising of prescription products. It would be helpful if there were more information on the Internet, not paid for by pharmaceutical companies, about the outcomes of treatments with various newer and expensive medications. For example, the NIH web site mentioned above has data for patients on newer classes of drugs for the lowering of cholesterol.

---

1. The vast web site of the NIH at http://www.nih.gov has links to health information for patients and health professionals.

Perhaps part of a national medical database for use by doctors and hospitals, and those gathering outcome data, would be a section for patients. There are huge savings in health care costs if an informed patient population learns to avoid expensive, marginally effective, or potentially harmful treatments with the use of information from online sources.

Of course, there is a lot of garbage online. A huge industry has sprung up to market "all-natural, non-toxic" alternative products. Some sellers of supplements have slick web sites, complete with references to scientific articles, and some of this material seems to include legitimate research results from respected sources. A new role for a primary care doctor is to help the patient sort through the information presented. These days, doctors who are at the cutting edge of technology have lists of web sites ready to hand to patients about particular health problems and may have Internet access in the office. Some information about prevention and treatment changes so rapidly that the Internet becomes the ideal source of centrally collected up-to-date treatment. An example is health information for travelers to developing nations. The web site of the Centers for Disease Control[2] has accurate and recent information on the prevention of malaria, yellow fever, dengue fever, and other tropical diseases. A doctor who glances at a patient's itinerary and downloads the pertinent information becomes much more effective at helping the patient get the right immunizations and preventative medications. Nonetheless, so many primary care doctors are still computer illiterate, pressed for time, and otherwise unmotivated to do the necessary work to plan for health needs for travel that it is most often up to the patient to collect the recommendations and tersely state them at the doctor's office. Learning to collect needed health information from the Internet is becoming as essential for adults as learning how to drive an automobile.

I am not an advocate of "do-it-yourself" medicine. Early in the 20th century, my wife's grandmother used the equipment in her sewing box to treat lacerations on the ranch in southern California. I hope that era will not be returning. Rather, a partnership between the patient and the doctor can produce the best result over the long run. Patients can gather some fairly technical data, but an experienced doctor is the best guide to using it.

---

2.   The web site of the Centers for Disease Control at http://www.cdc.gov/travel/ lists travel information by geographical area.

Solutions: Deregulation

When I abandoned my solo internal medical practice in 2001, a major factor contributing to my action was my being buried under a pile of regulations. Several hours of each busy day were consumed by paperwork that contributed nothing to the health of my patients. Many pieces of paperwork were generated by health insurers to slow the process of payment for services.

One source of copious paperwork and regulation is the federal government, in particular the agency overseeing Medicare, the primary insurance for so many of my older patients. This huge agency has been known as the Healthcare Financing Administration or HCFA, pronounced HICK-FEH in medical circles. However, by the time you read this, the new name for the agency, the Center for Medicare and Medicaid services or CMS, will have taken effect. I suspect that billions of dollars will be spent to implement the name change and modify all the forms to show the new appellation, but that is a separate issue from the problem of regulation as experienced by doctors and hospitals.

In an effort to reduce spending, a diagnosis-based fixed-fee schedule was introduced for hospitals in 1984 for Medicare patients. Instead of paying for hospital care by the day and by the item of service rendered, an elaborate system of fixed payment based on diagnostic category was introduced. Over the years since, myriad refinements have been made to this scheme. Armies of personnel, both at the hospital and at the offices of Medicare contractors, who administer payment, are required to determine appropriate payment for services. In the case of doctors, a fee schedule based on an elaborate series of numerical codes for services was established in 1984. Patients do not realize how tightly controlled the fee schedule is for Medicare with major penalties for violation of the charge limits. As of this writing, both hospitals and doctors are experiencing considerable fiscal stress due to 17 years of gradually lowering fees compared to the rising costs of doing business. The unfortunate results of fee control are the closing of hospitals and doctors leaving practice, events which are occurring with increasing frequency in the San Francisco Bay area where I practiced. For patients, finding a primary care doctor, who for adults is either a specialist in internal medicine or family practice, is becoming increasingly difficult. It is not simply the fees that are the problem for the doctors. The cost of compliance with all the numerous other Medicare regulations is quite significant. Every possible impediment to the smooth flow of patient care has been put in place for Medicare patients in an effort to save money. To order a simple lab test requires elaborate paperwork with the use of 5 digit numerical disease codes for each blood test. The diabetic needs monitoring of the disease, but without the correct code, 250.00 or whichever, the laboratory cannot collect the regulated fee of $3.25 for performing the test and a pile of paperwork is created when following up the deficiency in coding. Medicare has elaborate rules regarding the "medical necessity" of tests. "Screening" tests are not covered, with certain exceptions such as mammograms. Thus, the patient has to be diagnosed with a disease before the rules allow Medicare payment for tests to monitor it. In practice, there is a huge gray zone between screening and treating. For example, diabetic patients often have disturbances in cholesterol related to the metabolic problems caused by their disease. Is it screening or treating to test the cholesterol of a diabetic patient? I would contend that it is both. Medicare administrators could contend that it is a screening test, and accuse a doctor of "fraud and abuse" in ordering a cholesterol blood panel on a diabetic patient with unknown and perhaps normal cholesterol using a code such as 272.0 for elevated cholesterol. Yet, this happens thousands of times each day, as doctors try to take care of patients under difficult circumstances. Note that doctors generally do not own laboratories and do not profit from ordering laboratory testing, yet they are potentially liable for criminal action if they order a test that is deemed not medically necessary. There are elaborate paperwork procedures available to have the patient sign a special "Advanced Beneficiary Notice" form, in which the patient acknowledges that he has been informed that Medicare will not cover the cholesterol test because the doctor ordered it for screening purposes. The resulting confused patient becomes quite indignant later. A bill arrives from the laboratory for a very high, unregulated fee for the test, since it is no longer reimbursed under the tight Medicare fee schedule. Laboratories tend to "cost shift" to unregulated patient tests a very high fee to compensate for the very low fee schedules of Medicare and other insurers. Those who pay cash, have a self-insurance plan without contractually arranged discounts, or are paying for a non-covered screening test are charged many multiples of the rate on the Medicare fee schedule for covered services. In other words, the fees for many patients are deeply discounted by law or contract. For the few who pay the whole bill, the charges are much higher than a fair rate, as desperate hospitals, doctors, labs, and X-ray facilities attempt to compensate for falling income by charging whatever they can to the few who might pay the inflated "regular" charges. Any test done under the "not medically necessary" rule of Medicare is fair game for the higher, unregulated charges.

Somewhere among the government agencies and their contractors who control and perform the processing of claims for Medicare patients, vast sums of money are disappearing to administer these elaborate schemes of price control. Medicare is proud to quote a very low administrative overhead. I don't think anyone actually knows how many federal dollars disappear into the micromanagement of the care of Medicare patients, and the indirect costs in each doctor's office and at each hospital are huge. Yet the answer to the ever-rising costs of health care and ever-increasing outflows from the Medicare trust fund is to generate more controls and more regulations. I was already in the process of closing down my practice at the end of 2001 when a new 5.4 percent cutback for doctor's fees was announced for 2002. Those doctors who remain faced the rising cost of office space, employees, supplies, and insurance, while earning less and less per patient encounter. Soon, a 4.4 percent cutback for 2003 may be implemented.

As I will discuss in the next chapter, there is not enough money available for health care to provide everything for everyone, but the current cost-control schemes are creating a slow death for many institutions and doctors. Health care reform will require deregulation, not more controls. The failure of managed care is another part of the misguided effort to micromanage every aspect of patient care, only to have the cost of regulation exceed the savings and kill the doctors and the hospitals in the process. Professionals, operating autonomously, tend to do a good job and expect to earn a living performing their work. We now have an ailing profession in which good work is punished, and it is very difficult to earn a living. Many shrug their shoulders and angrily slog on, lengthening the work week, doing quick and shoddy patient care to compensate for the falling fees. When questioned about the state of their world, the answer is "I have no choice." We haven't yet measured the decline in the quality of health care delivered by downtrodden professionals, but there are many anecdotal reports of faltering performance. Unhappy doctors do slipshod work. The financially pressed hospitals thin out the nursing staffs to save money and the staffs are overworked, stressed, and prone to errors in patient care. The answer to alleged increases in mistakes in hospitals has been to pass new federal legislation and create new forms to fill out to report errors when they occur. This is exactly the opposite of what is needed, a reduction in paperwork or computerwork to allow more staff time at the patient bedside.

The key to cost savings, in my opinion, is to have highly trained, highly experienced doctors on the front lines of care. The front lines are the offices of doctors who are board certified in family practice, internal medicine, and pediatrics. These doctors are certified because they have completed a minimum of three years of training in one of these primary care specialties and have passed a Board exam certifying their knowledge. In the course of training they have cared for the sickest of the sick. They have lost much sleep, and have missed time with family and friends. They have dealt with the death of numerous patients and cared for the families of these patients. Each doctor has been present thousands of times for some of the worst events of people's lives. To be a doctor is to accept the ultimate accountability. You cannot turn around and look to a person behind you to make a decision for you. Yes, you can get an opinion from a subspecialist consultant, but the most effective and competent doctor lets it be known to patient, family, and consultant that he or she is the guiding force in the case.

If we want to reduce costs for the health care system as a whole, the energetic, talented primary care doctors on the front lines need to be unshackled from regulations, paper, and the burden of capitation. How will we know what kind of job they are doing? Would we be able to weed out impaired or incompetent doctors? Hopefully, with a national medical data base, aberrant patterns of care could be discerned and dealt with fairly, with efforts to educate and correct for minor deviations from expected performance.

Emergency rooms and hospitals are very expensive to operate and staff. So much of everyday health care can be provided in a doctor's office, with much lower costs per patient encounter. A seasoned primary care doctor can do 90 percent of the care of a patient 90 percent of the time, right out of a small office. The real savings to the health care system would come from deregulating and from rewarding good primary care, so that the brightest and best would be attracted to the primary care training programs and not clamor to be heart surgeons. Every attempt to save a fraction of the market-determined cost of primary care has produced an adverse fiscal effect, namely higher utilization of tests, hospitals, emergency rooms, and expensive subspecialty procedures. Every new form to fill out represents a waste of effort, energy, and money that should be directed at sick people, now. We can make better choices for using the training and experience of doctors.

Paradoxically, the crisis in accessibility to health care in the United States may lead to an increase in regulation. There are increasing calls for universal health care access under a single-payer plan, perhaps administered by Medicare. Recently, the head of a major insurance company, Bruce Bodaken of Blue Shield of California, called for universal health care.[1] He stated that "the current system and its underlying economics are unsustainable." His plan would involve the private sector by having required insurance, paid for by employers or the government, for everyone. A true single-payer plan would essentially put health insurers out of business, except perhaps as contractors to administer benefits as is done in the Medicare program.

The challenge is to preserve and enhance simple access to primary care for all citizens, and to promote restrained use of scarce resources while doing so. Canada's single-payer system provides comparatively simple access to primary care, but there are long lines[2] for high tech procedures. A parallel private system has been developing in some provinces, leading to calls for increased funding for the single-payer system.[3] Many Canadians have crossed the border into the United States to get high-tech procedures performed more quickly.

We have learned that *carte blanche* payment for all services by insurance leads to extreme overutilization and exponentially expanding health care costs. The answer to this problem has been ever-increasing regulations and paperwork. I hope that with an emphasis on strong primary care, an online data base of preferred treatment protocols for common diseases, and increasing understanding of the limits of technology, we will be able as a society to do much good for all citizens with the first 10 percent of health care dollars spent. Then we can go on to learn to use the expensive 90 percent of procedures more wisely.

1.   Appleby, J. Insurer wants universal health care. *USA Today*, December 4, 2002.
2.   Krauss, C. Long lines mar Canada's low-cost health care. *NY Times*, February 13,2003.
3.   Krauss, C. Canada's health care system needs more cash, panel says. *NY Times*, November 29, 2003.

Solutions: A Rational Approach to Rationing

A feature of the fast-paced 1990s was the prominence of political correctness in American culture. Certain ideologies became incorrect with a capital "I." Egalitarianism is politically correct. Discrimination is politically incorrect. Even as economic statistics revealed an increasing spread between the very rich and the very poor, public statements by politicians of both major parties always included caveats about making material wealth available to all Americans. The prosperity of the late 1990s produced euphoria about including all citizens in its benefits. Yet, at the same time, the continuing rise in health care costs and the effects of managed care and federal price controls were squeezing doctors and hospitals, in some cases to a slow, fiscal death. Most working people are well most of the time. Asking them to share in the very high cost of caring for the few who are sick during a period of economic prosperity does not produce a friendly outpouring of voluntary contributions. When well, employees and their families opt for the lowest cost health insurance available, if they have health insurance at all. They do not see themselves as part of the rising demand for health care services, and they do not view the rising costs of health care as their problem. One recent medical journal editorial[1] suggested that the cost squeeze on doctors and hospitals threatens the very existence of the health care system.

Despite the increasingly limited financial resources available to care for sick people, in the dot com boom era of the 1990s politicians were still issuing rhetoric about the need for universal basic health care. "Wonderful health care for every man, woman, and child, for less than we pay now" is a powerful campaign slogan. One word not seen in public statements was the "R" word, rationing. Rationing had become a forbidden word by the 1990s. Its dictionary definition, "to restrict to limited allotments," in no way suggests discrimination based on any personal or group traits. But in our culture, the word rationing now has

---

1. Sandy, LG. Homeostasis without reserve—the risk of health system collapse. *NEngl J Med 2002;* 347:1971-1975.

strong connotations of unequal distribution of goods and services. "That group over there gets more health services than this group over here." A very un-American scenario, yet even as it is forbidden to talk of rationing, the current serious maldistribution of health care services is *de facto* rationing, and it is getting worse. Aside from the tens of millions of people with no health insurance at all, access to care for those with a health plan is slowly worsening. One politician, who also happens to be an M.D., wasn't afraid to use the "R" word. Governor John Kitzhaber of Oregon initiated a storm of controversy with his plan to make use of limited Medicaid resources by allocating limited funds to just those medical conditions where the greatest benefit of treatment could be obtained for the most people. The original 1989 plan added many uninsured working poor to Medicaid in Oregon and paid for this expansion in the program by covering fewer services. In 1991, the Oregon state legislature ranked more than 700 diagnoses and treatments in order of importance. Medicaid would not cover treatments below item 587. Someone suffering from a rare neurological disorder might find his or her disease lower on the list and therefore not be eligible for Medicaid coverage of its treatment. Yet those who supported the Oregon plan for rationing limited health care resources found it one of the rare honest approaches to relating the use of limited funds to results. More people could get more treatment than if a few people had full coverage for every condition. Heart attacks were covered. Facial acne was not. The outcome of the first seven years of the Oregon Health Plan was reviewed in the New England Journal of Medicine.[2]

The image of the friendly general practitioner who knew everyone in the neighborhood and was available day and night for every little medical problem has evolved into something much less pleasant for the sick patient. Due to insurance restrictions, the patient must seek attention from an unfriendly medical group, with care available only after a long hold on the phone and a long wait to get an appointment. The professional providing the care may be a nurse or technician, not a doctor. To me, this is the rationing of care at its worst. Withholding services as much as possible is conserving limited resources, namely the capitation payments received by a medical group. More services are apportioned to those who whine and scream the loudest on the telephone. We have developed a health care system that rations care by discriminating against the polite and unassertive members of society. "Call back in two weeks if your cough is not any better. In

2.   Bodenheimer T. The Oregon Health Plan—lessons for the nation. First of two parts. *N Engl J Med* 1997;337(9):651-5, and
      Bodenheimer T. The Oregon Health Plan—lessons for the nation. Second of two parts. *N Engl J Med* 1997;337(10):720-3.

the meantime, take an over-the-counter cough medicine containing dextromethorphan." So the polite patient, hearing this standard advice from the phone receptionist, comes to the emergency room a few days later with pneumonia. The assertive patient who plaintively cries, "I can't breathe!" on the phone is seen on an urgent basis and is perhaps diagnosed with bronchitis or pneumonia before needing hospitalization.

Rationing in this way is occurring on the front lines of health care, the primary physician group offices. But it is also occurring in the specialist offices based on insurance coverage of the patient. Some invasive and potentially dangerous testing, like coronary angiography, is done sooner and more frequently on patients with better insurance. (Coronary angiography is a test performed by a cardiologist in which plastic tubes are inserted in a major blood vessel and threaded several feet into the heart. Dye is squirted to make the vital coronary arteries visible on X-ray. Blockages that lead to heart attack can be diagnosed and treated.)

The majority of coronary angiograms are performed on patients who need them rather desperately. They may have chest pain with exertion or an abnormal result on an exercise stress test. But there are numerous less urgent, somewhat marginal situations, in which the patient is stable, medication is working to stop chest pain, and there is no immediate life-threatening need to do the test. I have observed repeatedly in these cases that the better the insurance coverage, the more likely such a patient is to have a coronary angiogram or other invasive tests. If the patient has old-fashioned full-pay indemnity insurance, he or she is first in line; with a PPO, next; and with a capitated HMO plan, "Let's try this medication for another month, do another treadmill stress test on you heart, and see what the situation is then."

The scenario I have described is rationing in action as a result of managed care and very disparate payments for services under different insurance programs. It is ugly and discriminatory to differentiate the intensity of patient care in this way, yet it is an everyday reality. Subtle and not-so-subtle economic pressures influence medical decision making in thousands of offices, clinics, and hospitals across the United States. Maybe we really do have something to scream about.

But let us return for a moment to the golden age of the General Practitioner. Try to imagine a return to a world in which you and your family have a caring and readily available primary physician. In the present, he or she would no longer be a general practitioner, but might be an internist or family practitioner. Or the kids would see a pediatrician and the parents would see an internist. What would it take to bring back primary care to what we would like it to be? What would it cost to make it available to every American? Therein lies the problem. I have done a rough thumbnail calculation of the cost of health care per person if we were to make it available in an accessible and empathetic style to each person. My rough estimate of the cost for 2002 is *$1000 per month for every man, woman, and child in the United States.* This assumes that each person has equal access to good care and the total cost is distributed equally among all citizens on a per-month basis. Very few families could afford this type of expense on their own. To mandate that employers pay this amount of money on behalf of each employee and her or his dependents is not plausible. For the economically well versed, we are talking about a total cost equal to 30 percent of the gross domestic product for health care compared to the current 14 percent. Of course, we have more than 40 million uninsured Americans and another 60 million who get service only in the setting of a major emergency, and providing better coverage for these people under the current hodgepodge of federal and state programs might cost nearly as much.

Some people would argue, "Let the government pay for it!" Well, the government has paid for it already in the form of Medicare, Medicaid, and other programs. Actual utilization of services always exceeds the budget, and the resulting bureaucratic effort to contain costs destroys the flow of services that the program is supposed to provide. The inefficiencies built into any large government bureaucracy suck up much of the money allocated to patient care. Taxpayers do not receive the best value for their dollars when they bear the cost of health care through the collection of taxes and redistribution of the money into government health programs. The trend to capitated care in employer-based programs may not be any more efficient. Money disappears into the profit margin of the management company, into utilization review, quality assurance monitoring, and a dozen other administrative programs designed to monitor a type of financing for health services that is intrinsically disordered. Doctors and hospitals are paid *not* to treat under capitated HMO-type plans. After the results are noted to be less than optimum for the insured groups, more and more of the premium dollars are spent on making rules to assure that people get the services they are denied. To me, capitation is a chaotic, discriminatory system, rationing at its worst.

So, who is going to pay for health care? I do not have an easy answer. It never was easy, as the previous generation of GPs would testify. There were unpaid bills and plucked chickens left on the front seat of the doctor's car.

Making the patient pay the first couple of thousand dollars per year of costs and then a decreasing percentage of subsequent costs seems to make sense. People will wait a few extra days for their sore elbow to take care of itself if they have to bear the full expense of an office visit. But the patient with a devastating stroke and subsequent paralysis and disability is usually unable to bear the latter $80,000 of his or her $100,000 illness.

There may be a practical ceiling on employer contributions to employee health care insurance premiums. Perhaps the role of the federal government should be to contribute part of the premium for private insurance costs, with the decreasing deductible scheme helping to control utilization. This does not solve the problem of apportioning limited resources, and any federal involvement invariably leads to extra piles of paperwork. Perhaps with a national medical database, cost accounting and co-payment procedures could be drastically simplified and automated to allow smooth flow of care.

The other aspect of rationing is the need to apportion limited resources among those who benefit the most from them. An oversimplified example would be to say that a 45-year-old benefits more from a coronary bypass procedure than an 85-year-old, because they have longer to live. Society may benefit because the 45-year-old will go back to work and contribute back to society in taxes apportioned to health care more than the cost of the bypass procedure. The 85-year-old has long since retired. On the surface, it appears that we are allocating limited resources by discriminating on the basis of age and material contribution to society, ranking people on a scale of social worth. But actually, the situation is much more complex.

There are overriding health considerations in deciding whether or not to do a coronary bypass procedure on an 85-year-old that have nothing to do with the cost. The majority of bypass procedures are performed by placing the patient on bypass; that is, stopping the heart and pumping the blood through a machine to oxygenate it. Brain damage is common during this procedure, even in the most experienced hands. Approximately 10 percent of patients over 80 have a stroke during the procedure, which in some cases can be permanently disabling. Another 10-20 percent suffer a more subtle form of brain damage that may not be noticed until weeks later. There is impairment of memory and perhaps control of movement in a subtle way, but this too can be disabling. The bypass has been technically successful, the patient will not die of a heart attack in the next 15 years, but he can't remember names, numbers, and events like he used to, and his balance is impaired so he falls over while teeing off on the golf course.

It takes considerable training and experience to help a patient and family make an informed decision about whether or not to proceed with a bypass procedure. There are alternative treatments available. Medication can stop the chest pain and allow the continuation of most daily activities. Balloon angioplasty can often open up the most critically blocked of multiple diseased coronary arteries, reducing the more imminent threat of a major heart attack. The heart surgeon might argue that the angioplasty is a temporary measure and not a cure, but is this a relevant point? To the 85-year-old, if an angioplasty stops the pain and he is recovered from that procedure in two days, is there a need for worry about the remaining partially blocked vessels? These might cause trouble a couple of years down the road, or another disease may be more of a problem by then. On the other hand, the 45-year-old might do better getting all seven blockages in his heart fixed with a bypass, including the six that are not imminently life threatening. He will likely recover much faster than the 85-year-old, and the concept of "surgical cure" is appealing to someone who plans to be working and active for the next 20 years. To do the bypass on the 45-year-old and not on the 85-year-old might just be good medicine rather than discrimination on the basis of age.

In the decision-making process, there are a number of other non-financial considerations. There is the concept of co-morbidity. A simple example would be the patient with a terminal cancer who develops chest pain. Life expectancy is short, a matter of months, and medication can be used to stop the chest pain. Heart catheterization, angioplasty, and bypass seem irrelevant for the heart disease in this patient who is in a terminal phase of an untreatable cancer.

What about a 70-year-old with early Alzheimer's disease, who might live another eight years with a gradual decline in memory and ability to do self-care? If this patient develops chest pain with minimal exertion and has an abnormal electrocardiogram, how far should he be taken down the cascade from catheterization and angiography to angioplasty to bypass? "Well, he is still walking around, living with his family," notes the cardiologist. After the angiogram reveals a life-threatening blockage to a main coronary artery that cannot be ballooned open, the heart surgeon says, "I can bypass this patient in under 90 minutes and he'll be home walking around in a week." But the patient's mental status can actually deteriorate markedly after a bypass, making him less independent and more disabled. As his primary care internist muttered, "There are fates worse than death."

So many of the invasive, expensive, painful procedures done on elderly patients have a very marginal benefit, especially when you consider the outcome over time for a large group undergoing the procedure. Gathering the data on outcomes is hampered by our lack of a central repository for health data and may be hampered further by the new federal privacy legislation. The best ally for the family is an experienced primary doctor who knows the patient and can put the pros and cons of doing the procedure in perspective for the patient and family. It takes training and experience to have the skill to be an advocate for what is best for the patient. To the cardiologist, the pressure is on to do the heart catheterization and get on with the next case. To the heart surgeon, the world can be defined simply: "A chance to cut is a chance to cure." It is easy to do a good surgery, technically perfect, and have a bad outcome that is a problem for the patient but not for the surgeon. "You are recovered from your bypass now. I hope your dizziness goes away. It can happen to patients on the pump. I have nothing more to offer. Go see your internist." The patient begins to realize that he might have been slightly better off with no surgery at all.

Unfortunately, we are moving away from making careful decisions about treatment. The internist or family doctor may be nowhere in sight in the hospital, the hospital care delegated to the specialists in an effort to crank out more patient volume in the office. There is no time for the extra care in mulling over the pros and cons of a procedure. The patient is having chest pain and the catheterization is performed. If anything, the decision-making process is simplified to a cookbook-style recipe. Thinking takes time. Time is money. There is less and less money per patient and per procedure in the system. Some money remains for procedures. Almost no money remains for thinking. This is the nuts and bolts of an ailing health care system and a medical profession in decline. We have reduced a major life decision to a wham-bam, no-think, and just-do-it simplified process. Adverse results may be far more costly than the price of the procedure, but these costs occur later, outside the hospital, spread over time. They do not affect the accounting for the HMO or PPO benefits of the patient in the hospital.

We can improve this situation immensely because we have a supply of talented and experienced primary care doctors in the specialties of internal medicine and family practice, who need to be adequately paid to take a strong role in the major decisions in the hospital. They know the patient. They can weigh the effect of other diseases and problems on the outcome of a proposed major procedure. They know how the patient's diabetes might affect the situation. They know of the elderly patient's wishes not to have artificial life support. Without the guidance of a strong, primary M.D., the patient cruises through the hospital on autopilot, scribbling a signature on the required consent forms without understanding what is being signed. "Everyone gets everything." The "everything" is a pile of extremely expensive procedures, ranging from life saving to very marginally useful, many with long-term consequences that are negative.

In promoting a "rational approach to rationing," I am talking about using limited resources wisely and with restraint based on a broad view of all the possible outcomes. I champion the involvement of the primary care doctor in these decisions. They are not discriminatory based on age or prior disability. The decision process takes into account the potential for benefit and the potential risks and long-term negative results of the procedure. There are quality of life issues that need to be considered based on the patient's preferences rather than the narrow view of the specialist performing the procedure. In quieter times in the office, it is the duty of the primary care doctor to discuss contingency plans with the patient in the event of life-threatening illness. Many patients have watched loved ones and acquaintances go through a long downhill course, lengthened by painful and aggressive interventions in the hospital that did not produce an improvement in the quality of life. As these patients get older, they may say, "Take care of the small things Doc, and keep me going, but if something bad happens, just keep me comfortable." Most states in the U.S. have codified this request into a formal "Advanced Directive for Health Care" or "Living Will"-type of document. Discussing these documents and even providing the blank forms are important duties of the primary care doctor. They should not be delegated to a social worker at the hospital whom the patient does not know and discussed when the patient is ill, anxious, on pain medication, and unable to think clearly. The time to think about such difficult issues as life support is before the patient needs it, not while she or he is lying semi-comatose in the emergency room. In caring for people as they age over a period of many years, those of us who have been primary care doctors for elders develop a sense of the cycle of life. We begin to discern at a subtle level which problems can be helped by medical technology and for which problems the available treatment is worse than the disease. Perspective comes with time and experience. Many patients develop perspective as they go through life. Should they not have a caring doctor who also has perspective?

Perhaps we will someday have a national medical database in which medical researchers can access anonymously the long-term consequences of particular procedures. We might move closer to the Truth with a capital "T" about the merits of a particular piece of technology. Until then, there is a strong subjective element, the art of medicine, that needs to be applied carefully to each patient. A long-term relationship with an experienced primary care M.D., unfettered by relationships to managed care companies or government agencies, provides the patient with the best chance for optimal results from treatment at the lowest possible cost. Intrinsic to the primary care role is the development of great skill in knowing when to send the patient down a high-tech, costly, specialist-treatment cascade, and when simple comfort measures will suffice. This may be "rationing," but we don't think of it that way. I would call it "good care."

What You Should Do Now as a Patient

If you have found yourself unable to get health care easily in an urgent situation or if you have spent hours waiting in an emergency room for treatment of an urgent but non-life-threatening illness or injury, you know firsthand about the decline in American medicine.

To have the best possible outcome for your health, you need to stay educated, consider options to improve your access to care, and voice your concerns to your Human Resources Department, to government officials, and to your insurer. Also, become aware of the Advanced Directives for Health Care available in your state. Let us look briefly at each of these areas.

Staying educated about treatment guidelines and screening for common diseases is essential for every patient. Patients need to be involved in, and take responsibility for, all aspects of their health care. For many of us, gone are the days when a reminder card comes from a doctor's office telling us it was time for an annual physical exam or a periodic screening test. Especially in the era of capitated care, there are financial rewards for allowing physical exams to slide and, along with them, the schedule of annual screening procedures. If your health plan does encourage you to receive annual screening procedures, a nurse or technician who does not know you may perform them as part of a mass screening program, during which you line up with dozens of other patients and go through the screening in assembly-line fashion. The press is filled with the stories of patients whose abnormal results fell through the cracks until it was too late. In automated mass screening programs, a simple error in an address or phone number may make contacting the patient about abnormalities impossible.

If you are caring for children, make sure you are up-to-date on the recommendations for immunizations. A search of the Internet under the heading "Immunization Schedule" will bring you up-to-date information on recommendations from the Centers for Disease Control[1] and other agencies. Some newer immuni-

---

1. http://www.cdc.gov/nip/

zations are very costly, and health plans are slow to adopt reimbursement for them as a benefit for plan members. An example is the newer hepatitis vaccines. It has become the responsibility of the parents to learn which vaccines are required and aggressively pursue obtaining them.

As an adult, you need to educate yourself about the major risk factors for atherosclerosis, or hardening of the arteries, a disease that ultimately affects half of us. Some of the risk factors include high blood pressure, elevated cholesterol, diabetes, cigarette smoking, and a family history of heart attacks and strokes in parents and grandparents. The web site at the National Institutes of Health[2] contains a wealth of information on this subject. It is useful for each adult to set up a file at home for him- or herself, and get copies of screening results, such as lab tests for cholesterol and serial blood pressure readings, and keep these for future use. So many males of working age ignore risk factors for atherosclerosis until they find themselves in the emergency room with their first heart attack. Good preventative care for coronary disease is available but is most useful if started 20 years before the first clogged-artery event.

The other major class of disease, affecting nearly one in three of us, is cancer. There are many do-it-yourself screens, such as for melanoma, and a list of recommended tests from Pap smears to prostate antigens. These are described in another portion of the vast National Institutes of Health web site, starting at the National Cancer Institute information page.[3] Once again, I recommend getting copies of cancer screening test results for your own file. Frequent shifts in health plans may result in sudden changes in your "designated" doctor and hospital, and the instability in the health care system results in frequent changes in practice location for many doctors. Few of us will have the same friendly doctor for decades, and increasingly patients are "on their own" in seeking and obtaining well-person screening and even in interpreting the results.

What is the best source of general medical information for the lay person? I have mentioned sources on the Internet for information on immunizations, atherosclerosis, and cancer, but there are many everyday symptoms for which access to professional care is a major hassle and self-treatment may be the best or only option. A number of university medical centers publish health newsletters or "wellness" newsletters for the general public. Subscribing to one of these allows one to keep up with disease treatments, including self-treatments, for a variety of ailments. There are also a number of health encyclopedia type publications,

---

2.   http://www.nhlbi.nih.gov/
3.   http://www.cancer.gov/cancer_information/

although these tend to go out-of-date rather quickly. Non-profit organizations publish useful newsletters for particular diseases, such as arthritis or Parkinsonism. Your local Health System may sponsor classes at relatively low cost about such issues as Women's Health and Well Baby Care. There are also many questionable sources of health information available, often linked to the sale of vitamins or other products purported to provide an alternative treatment for troubling symptoms. As a general rule, publications that offer knowledge, not products, are a more reputable source of health information.

Options to improve access to care include changing insurance plans. In this first decade of the new millennium, employers are shifting more of the burden for health insurance premiums onto employees. Usually, an HMO-type plan with relatively poor access to care has a much lower paycheck deduction than a PPO-type plan with better access. Few families have access to an old-fashioned indemnity plan with complete choice of doctors and hospitals. It is often difficult to determine the type of plan from its name. Insurance companies long ago learned to hide the term HMO and the fact that a plan turns the patient into a "capitated life," a dehumanized entity that the health care system tries to ignore as much as possible.

There is a new expensive option for health care access springing up around the United States: "boutique"-style primary care practices in which the patient pays an annual retainer fee to cover the cost of good phone access to the doctor and timely responses to patient needs. The retainer can range from $1500 to $5000 per year. In addition, patients are expected to pay the full cost of all office services and do their own insurance billing, usually recouping only a fraction of the fees. Government agencies have been investigating methods to stop this practice, alleging that it is discriminatory based on the income level of the patient. It is likely that "boutique" care, unreimbursed by government or private insurance also threatens to derail the micromanagement goals of the government and insurance industry bureaucracies that I have described in this book. However, it is possible to imagine a new form of insurance with a very high annual deductible and a shrinking co-payment as the patient requires more services, which would mesh with this new style of practice and make it more affordable to working people.

This discussion of new options outside the existing insurance system leads to the last point, namely that patients have to make noise, even when they are healthy and not utilizing many health services. They need to talk to the people responsible for selecting the choices of health plans for their employer, usually in the Human Resources Department, and inform them of the deterioration in care. They need to complain to the insurer or managed care companies when care is inadequate or delayed. And they need to send letters or e-mail to their Senators and Congressperson telling them of the problems encountered in obtaining health care, and of the need to modify the provisions of ERISA to allow third-party benefit administrators, HMOs, and insurers to share the liability for bad health outcomes.

The latest news on declining access to health care is a new forecast[4] for a shortage of physicians in the U.S. For 20 years, predictions have been for a glut of doctors. Warnings by economists that the surplus would lead to increased health expenditures and produce negative effects on the entire economy have filled medical and health policy journals. We are just now entering the phase of public awareness of a doctor shortage. The economists still push for the substitution of primary care doctors with nurse practitioners, citing tremendous cost savings. They are more worried that the cardiologists and other vital subspecialists will be in short supply. As I have argued throughout this book, the greatest cost savings can be achieved by having outstanding primary care internists, pediatricians, and family practitioners readily available for acute medical problems. The best outcome in changing poor lifestyle habits is the presence of a concerned M.D. who knows the patient over the long-term. The never-ending struggle to control health care costs will likely throw out the baby with the bath water once again, missing the opportunity to reduce the utilization of extremely expensive, high-tech, ultra specialized procedures too late in the course of a disease.

For seniors, the problem is particularly difficult. As people get older and sicker, the care of a diligent and experienced internist or family physician is needed to help treat deterioration in multiple body functions. Even with Medicare Part A and Part B coverage, access to a primary physician is difficult in many parts of the U.S. One study demonstrated increased frequency of hospitalization among elderly patients with poor health in areas where supply of primary care doctors is low.[5]

Access to health care and quality of health care may have to deteriorate further before a major national crisis is declared and changes are made. Until then, stay involved, stay informed, and exercise the available choices to try to get the best for yourself and your family. And try to imagine having a wonderful general doctor, who actually returns your phone calls and provides care the day you need it. If you are fortunate enough to have an accessible caring "provider," even a doctor substitute, mention your concern about Advance Directives for Health Care. The

---

4.   http://www.ama-assn.org/sci-pubs/amnews/pick_02/prl20121.htm
5.   http://archfami.ama-assn.org/issues/v8n6/ffull/foc8033.html

time to discuss your preferences for aggressive treatment of life-threatening illness is when you are well, not when you are lying on a stretcher in the emergency room. Would you want to be kept alive with machines to breathe for you and tubes to feed you, when there was little hope for a meaningful recovery? As people get older, some prefer to have "everything" done in the event of serious illness. Many others only want to be kept comfortable if there is little hope of recovery of independent living and normal daily activities. The sad reality of the current state of medical technology is that we are able to keep people alive sicker longer, rather than make them well. The idea of a "complete cure" through a high-tech procedure is mostly a fantasy. You need only to take a walk through the nearest skilled nursing facility in your area to see a collection of the people for whom medical technology has been a failure. No one wants to spend some of their last days or months (or years!) in a nursing facility, yet statistics show that *nearly one in two of us* will have that experience.

The time to dwell on the misery of chronic disability and dependence on others for feeding, toileting, and even turning over in bed is long before you are in that state. At least you should put some thought into the unpleasant subject and try to talk about it with a primary doctor sufficiently to be able to execute an advanced directive for health care and keep it on file. For each person, there can be a boundary delineating which kinds of aggressive treatment are appropriate and which ones should not be offered. Civil libertarians might decry my recommendations as discriminatory or potentially discriminatory based on age or disability, but I do not mean to use any one demographic trait as the final arbiter of the decision of whether to utilize artificial life support. The ultimate criterion in helping others to make a decision is a simple and human one: "What would you want for yourself or your loved ones in a similar situation?" We need to get that kind of personal, caring input from doctors into all encounters with very sick people. With the decline in the accessibility and concern of primary care doctors, it is not always there. What should we do to restore excellence in primary care?

Toward a New Medical Humanism

Some might hope that I would champion mandating free health care for all, paid for by someone else and provided by loving doctors who volunteer their services 24 hours per day. But I think that my view of instilling a humanistic tone and excellence in primary care, into the medical profession is somewhat more practical.

I have been lamenting the loss of control over one's professional life by each doctor and nurse and other caring providers of health services. The problem of too much demand for care paid for by increasingly strangling third parties has caused layers of Machiavellian regulations and paperwork to be placed between the sick patient and someone who can help him out now, today.

The human touch backed by professional knowledge has a value, and one aspect of that value is its worth in dollars at current market prices. When we remove the motivator and the barrier of market pricing for a particular service, we produce a gap between the supply and the demand for the service. Throughout history, regulation of prices has resulted in an unofficial, unregulated black market for the regulated items. If the item is an office visit, right now, today, needed desperately by a patient with a painful urinary tract infection, there is a market value for that service. It might be $100, and that may be well worth it to the patient suffering the condition. If the patient has to pay the amount out of her or his own pocket, some might find the $100 too expensive and choose to drink copious fluids and "flush out" the infection. Folk remedies, like cranberry juice extract, might be self-administered. Urinary tract infections often go away in a few days without professional treatment using these methods or without any treatment at all. When, under the current health insurance structure, the doctor is penalized financially for seeing the patient, he may try to treat the urinary infection by phone. Or, he may induce the patient to go somewhere else. Care and caring deteriorate when the health system is altered to provide financial disincentives to not see the patient.

Price controls, even with the maintenance of a fee-for-service structure, are also detrimental. If we make rules that the doctor can charge only $42 for care of the urinary tract infection, he may still try to see all patients with urinary tract infections out of a sense of professional duty and caring. He may have to shorten the visits, delegate them to a non-M.D. substitute, or see the patient in a less timely fashion. The waiting room may be packed at the doctor's office as an effort is made to "make up on volume" what has been lost by low, regulated fees. If we create a giant agency to oversee the prices of medical services, the initial success at budget control stimulates additional efforts to reduce utilization of medical services. It is possible to reduce the fees to a point at which care becomes scarce and the patient with symptoms is willing to pay much greater fees to be seen in the emergency room, where the treatment of a simple urinary tract infection is a $900 illness.

My experience in medical school was that the vast majority of students were highly idealistic and not motivated in their studies by the promise of future material gain. They were interested in science and people and were selected for these interests, along with excellence in academic achievement. They were in the middle of the12 years of study and training following high school that are necessary to produce a doctor ready to start practice. Most were living on student budgets. Few were concerned with making money. Yet, it was assumed that long years of effort would eventually result in a comfortable lifestyle. Now, with the slow collapse of the university medical schools, we have a generation of students who enter the profession with a huge burden of debt, as I have discussed previously. The rate of default on medical school debt has increased tremendously. Many doctors are not earning enough to make the loan payments.

There are many rewards in the practice of medicine outside of the payment for services provided. A dean in my medical school told us, as we started clinical rotations at the hospital, "The physician sees the patient into the world, and is there as the patient leaves the world." This was the role of the doctor in the era of the GP. We should bring back the doctor's professional role of "being there" for the patient and with the patient. The important moments of "being there" have been delegated to nurse-midwives, nurse practitioners, social workers, and physical therapists. These people are wonderful professionals (as I can attest after receiving physical therapy for a bad knee), but we should not expect them to be expert at the broad scope of treatment that the doctor acquires. The prestige of the profession and the art of healing depend on bringing back a strong and single identifiable primary care doctor for the patient, rather than a team of interchangeable substitutes, none of whom seem to really be in charge. A dwindling percentage of the population has had the experience of a caring doctor who shows concern for the whole person. There is clearly a demand for this type of service. Some of this style of practice has been incorporated into the practices of "alternative" and "holistic" practitioners. The growing numbers of patients seeking this mixture of mainstream and controversial medicine attests to what has been lost in the primary care specialties. If the mainstream health care delivery system no longer provides affable, affordable, accessible care when needed, people will seek any source that provides attention and concern.

No matter how idealistic, people-oriented, and motivated a young doctor may be, there needs to be some compensation for the considerable sacrifice one makes while training to be a doctor. What a doctor *should* earn is a subject that can be debated *ad nauseum*. I find it interesting to compare the salaries of doctors and baseball stars. In the late 1950s, a busy GP earned about the same amount of money as a superstar like Mickey Mantle. In 2001, superstar Derek Jeter was earning at least 250 times the annual income of a busy primary care doctor. Clearly, we have some extreme cycles in the relative value of different kinds of work.

In the era of the General Practitioner, there was little regulation of medical practice and fees were set more or less by market forces. There was a professional tradition of caring for those who could not pay. We have gone to such an opposite extreme, with total management of the fee structure by third parties and with such layers of microregulation, that we have stifled professionalism. I use "professionalism" to describe knowing the patients and their families, being available for crises large and small, and feeling fortunate to have the opportunity to be of help to sick people, and being willing to treat those who cannot pay for it. These very human professional traits have taken a downturn along with the self-esteem, income, satisfaction, and performance. I have witnessed the conversion of proud and caring professionals to "dweebs," where the goal is to get through hours of patient visits and paperwork as quickly as possible with as little emotion and patient interaction as possible. In many cases, this behavior has become necessary for economic survival. I am sure that health outcomes suffer under this type of care and long-term costs rise as minor conditions are ignored. The patient gets attention only when he rolls into the emergency room in a more advanced stage of his illness. There is no time in the office for the extra effort at disease prevention, and no time or interest in discussing future contingencies like the use of Advanced Directives for Health Care or Living Wills.

I have mentioned the "gray" market for caring services springing up in some areas of the U.S. The patient pays an annual retainer of several thousand dollars per year and agrees to pay a full price for office services outside of insurance restrictions, in return for access to the doctor via cell phone and digital messaging service 24 hours a day. It has been difficult to totally eliminate market forces, even with the mammoth effort by the federal government and private insurers to control fees.

But for the mainstream of medical practice these days, it is an increasingly oppressive effort to "make up on volume" what the doctor is not earning with the low and controlled fees. Along with what I call "dweebization" of the individual doctor comes the fall in self-esteem and income that leads many doctors to drop out of professional organizations. The excuse is that it is no longer easy to afford the annual dues. The combined annual membership dues in a county medical association, state medical association, and the American Medical Association can exceed $1000 per year. But a feeling of helplessness and hopelessness contributes to the decline in participation in organized medicine. I am reminded of Benjamin Franklin's statement at the signing of the Declaration of Independence, July 4, 1776, "We must all hang together, or assuredly we shall all hang separately." And indeed, there are many fine doctors out there twisting in the wind. Membership in the American Medical Association has fallen below 25 percent of the population of practicing doctors. As one politically involved doctor told me, the result of declining membership is declining influence in crafting legislation at the state and federal levels. He cited the Golden Rule of government, "Those with the gold make the rules." Right now, the rules are being made by the insurance and health management industry and their lobbyists, by the pharmaceutical industry, the hospital associations, consumer groups, and human rights organizations seeking more rules to benefit the disabled and to assure privacy of medical information.

To bring back the humanistic qualities to the profession, we will have to reward the behaviors that are admirable and once again allow market forces to regulate the price of the smaller everyday interactions with primary care doctors. The infrastructure is still there for the training of M.D.s in the primary care specialties of family practice, internal medicine, and pediatrics. It will be hard to find good role models for the trainees in these specialties because there are so few generalists who can afford the time to teach. The majority of full-time academicians, salaried by the medical schools, are subspecialists, expert in only one organ system of the body and ill-equipped to impart the values of the generalists to students. The hierarchy at medical schools rewards research and publication, not patient care and the teaching of medical students, and certainly not good care of an infected hangnail.

When I was teaching part time at a medical school-affiliated hospital in the 1980s, I watched the program director blast a resident in Internal Medicine for not having the time to look up an obscure disease presented at rounds the previous day. In the standard mode of hazing the resident (some would call it verbal abuse), the director screamed abrasively "If you are a good resident, I will get you into the best subspecialty fellowship! Otherwise, you can go be a GP!" In other words, poorly motivated trainees ran the risk of ending up as the lowest form of life, the generalist. The high achievers would follow their residency with more years of training in prestigious subspecialties like cardiology and gastroenterology and spend their days doing higher paid, high-tech procedures on sedated patients.

Some patients would define the humanistic quality of a doctor as "having a good bedside manner." Learning bedside manners started for me in the second year of medical school, in the first clinical course of the curriculum, as we began to learn patient interviewing and physical diagnosis techniques. A group of four students was introduced to patient care by watching a skilled and experienced doctor interview a selected, and quite verbal, patient, taking a medical history leisurely over an hour and a half. Our teacher wanted to show us how to leave no stone unturned in taking the history, to explore every subtlety of the patient's family and personal history, seeking clues to life stresses that had led to the current illness and hospitalization. Subsequently, we went on to do our own medical histories and physical exams on patients. Initially, the process took two or three hours, as we were all inept at the techniques. Positioning and inflating a blood pressure cuff could take 10 minutes. Later in medical school and residency, we learned to do a fairly complete case history and exam in 45 minutes, even faster under combat conditions when multiple critically ill patients needed our attention simultaneously.

Instilled in me by my teachers was a respect for the patient's pain and fear. Seriously ill people in a hospital are having a peak negative experience in their life. If the doctor is able to show focus and concern while doing a routine and perhaps dull series of steps in taking a history and doing the exam, it is a healing event for the patient. So many patients, struck down with a heart attack or collapsed with an overwhelming pneumonia and rolled into the hospital in a horizontal position, report later that "I started feeling better as soon as I got in here." The simple actions of nurses taking vital signs and asking about medications and allergies and the initial question by the doctor "What happened to you today?" have a very therapeutic effect. The fearful resignation to the feeling that "I am going to die today" is replaced by hope, as helpful, concerned, and knowledge-able people seem to be doing something about a personal disaster.

In the era during which the GP dominated the delivery of medical care, the help and the hope was in the hands of a single god-like figure who might have appeared in your bedroom at 2 AM. It was a time of paternalistic and comfort-oriented care, without the expensive technology of today's hospital. Patients were passive recipients of care, not participants in medical decision making. However, the majority of people, now over age 50, who recall that era, realize the values that have been lost as we have moved towards a technology-based, overly special-ized, bureaucratized system of health care. How much better are the outcomes in this new age? Well, we have added several years to the life expectancy of an American born today compared to that of an American born in 1950. But what is the quality of life in those extra years?

My observation is that we have failed to make *living* better in the extra years that the health care system and the medical profession have provided for the aver-age person. All of the expensive technology has failed us. I watched as a 70 year old man was snatched from the jaws of death by a cardiologist performing a bal-loon angioplasty and stent placement on a blocked coronary artery, only to see that patient have a devastating stroke six months later. He then spent three miser-able years in a nursing facility, half-paralyzed, unable to speak and passively hop-ing for oblivion to relieve his suffering. The subspecialists are nowhere to be seen once the patient is permanently committed to serving out his time in the nursing facility. The statistics on quality of care have chalked up another interventional cardiologist procedural success for the angioplasty. The $40,000 worth of doctor and hospital bills have been paid, albeit at a contractually reduced rate, by Medi-care and supplementary insurance. Now the patient's family is bearing the bur-den of the cost of chronic care in the nursing facility. The paralyzed man is generating bills of $5500 per month, and Medicare does not cover chronic custo-dial care in the nursing home. The new high-tech interventions are covered, but the real drain on family resources that occurs in chronic, disabling, slow-death kind of illness is not covered. The only exception is the coverage of Hospice care when a patient is in the last six months of a chronic downhill course from cancer or other disease, and the major benefits of Hospice occur if care can be provided in the home setting. But our patient is in a cramped two-bed room in a nursing facility, unable to even ring the call bell when he has soiled himself in his bed.

I have watched thousands of patients enter a final downhill cascade, a condi-tion of the entire person not evident when focusing only on a current crisis in one part of the body. The new technology fixes the heart with a bypass surgery, so now the patient lives to fall and break a hip. The smashed hip requires a big surgery for replacement of the ball and socket with a stainless steel prosthesis by an orthopedic surgeon. Several months of rehabilitation are required before the patient is able to care for himself or herself at home independently. The patient's memory is not as sharp as before, and a fancy array of neurological tests reveal that subtle brain damage occurred during the bypass surgery, rendering the patient unable to drive and somewhat forgetful. And then a slow and difficult course with a cancer begins...Several years later, the family is gathered at the memorial service, and one of the children comments, "It has been like one long illness for five years. We thought that the bypass would fix everything, but that was just the beginning of the sickness."

If the family was fortunate, there was a primary physician who actually followed the patient for the five years of illness. Having a primary doctor there, at least in the background, for all the crises, would have been a source of some words of perspective and some help getting a feeling of closure about the illness and death. But most families are on their own, with a sense of frustration that Dad or Mom "had to go through all of that." Imagine if there were a strong family doctor figure, caring also for the next generation of the family, who could channel some of the frustration about the loss into practical concern for the health of the sons and daughters of the patient. The downhill cascade for the patient started with heart disease and the bypass surgery, but the underlying hardening of the arteries started decades before. The sons and daughters of the deceased patient need to have their blood pressure and cholesterol checked, since these risk factors are commonly inherited from one's parents. The better use of health care dollars, compared to bypass surgery in the elderly, is the treatment of the risk factors in young and middle-aged adults.

Without availability and affordability of care and lacking the strong primary doctor role to encourage adherence to treatment regimes, prevention does not happen. By washing out the humanistic aspect to health care and by deemphasizing primary care, a greater and greater percentage of the population first gets care for heart disease when entering the health system via the emergency room, needing an immediate angioplasty or a bypass. In the broad view of the health care system and health care costs, that is a failure. These failures are costly and produce great suffering, but they make for spectacular TV serials about the emergency room and the hospital. The real caring and healing is less dramatic, much less expensive, and occurs quietly in the office of a primary care doctor. Follow-up office visits to recheck weight, blood pressure, and cholesterol and to encourage improvement in diet and exercise do not win TV drama awards. But as we decimate primary care doctors and drive them into shutting down their practices, prevention doesn't happen.

To the health policy makers, such failure to preempt disease 10 years before a crisis is difficult to measure and is therefore irrelevant. The cost savings for this year's budget for health care take precedence. Why not have a less expensive nurse or dietician follow the patient with risk factors for heart attack? Why pay more for the services of the doctor? The policy makers do not see the big picture over many years. They are unaware of the added value of regular contact with the professional who has the most training and the most experience. The doctor is the one whose ideal is to handle the whole patient, mind and body, all the organ systems, and to understand the long-term issues in health, not just the cholesterol reading of 342.

We have reached the point in my area of California at which, for many patients, some very routine, non-urgent issues are no longer addressed in an office. My emergency room doctor colleagues report the initiation of treatment for blood pressure and cholesterol problems simply because they felt it would have important long-term benefit and the patient was unable to get care elsewhere for these heart disease risk factors.

What a sorry state we have fallen into! Not only can the patient not get care for an uncomplicated sprained ankle today, in an office, for a reasonable charge. The whole health care system is so hobbled by inverted fiscal incentives not to treat, and by suffocating microregulation that the patient has difficulty obtaining the most obvious preventative measures for reducing the risk of future illness and disability. Let us bring back the caring primary doctor, someone who has spent years learning the art of caring for patients from birth to death. It does not matter whether the doctor's specialty is called "family practice" or "internal medicine" or something else. The point is that the art of caring for patients and families over the long haul has tremendous benefits in quality of care, accessibility of care, and reduction of costs. This care does not happen when fee schedules are restricted for the primary physician or capitated payments provide a fixed fee per month for not taking care of the patient.

I see around me the burnt-out remnants of professionals. What of those qualities we all hoped to have, or would hope to see in our own doctor? Qualities like grace, humility, reverence for the human body, knowledge of literature and music, and some sign of a joy of living. What have we become? Was it greed, unfulfilled expectations, and too much work with not enough fun that left us empty? Maybe some of the desirable qualities will return as the century long cycle of the medical profession reaches its bottom and starts upward again.

Closing Down the Practice: 2001

It is the last day. The office is largely empty now. My remaining loyal employee, office manager, and do-everything gal, has unplugged the last computer and I have carried it to the trunk of her car. She has agreed to do the last bits of bookkeeping out of her home. We lock the door and give the keys to the secretary of the new occupants. My office will no longer be a place to see patients; rather it will be the billing office for a large group of allergists. The office next door office used to have an internist; now it houses an "Appearance Enhancement Center." Two doors down, where there used to be a neurosurgeon, there is now a "Pain Management Center."

I had carefully crafted the timetable for shutting down my medical practice starting more than a year before the actual closure. A young colleague in the area agreed to take the patient records and many of the patients. There were documents to be drawn up and reviewed by the lawyers and a vast quantity of equipment to be disposed of. All kinds of business records had to be carefully sorted, boxed, and stored. Most importantly, patients had to be notified well in advance of the closing date and efforts made to have a seamless transition of their care to another doctor.

The announcement of my retirement from practice brought forth an emotional reaction from loyal patients. I was "too young to retire," they pleaded. I tried to explain how I had been buried by paperwork, my fees were regulated, and the expenses of running an office were still soaring. Many were unable to understand. "Doctors are rich!" "He made his millions off of us, and now he is going to sit back with his feet up."

In this book I have tried to explain why Michael Rosenblum, M.D., is no longer practicing internal medicine out of a solo office in Walnut Creek, California. Also, I have attempted to delineate the forces reducing the availability and quality of medical care for Americans, even in the face of spectacular advances in technology. I have presented some suggestions for improving access to care and quality of care, with the goal of long-term cost savings as well.

I feel a sense of loss, not seeing patients, for there is great satisfaction in trying to help with the miseries of sickness and age. I sit at the computer terminal, typing this manuscript. When the words no longer bubble up into awareness, I put on my boots and dig in my steep hillside garden. The world below me seems peaceful and well, and after a little while, the words return.

0-595-28419-1

Printed in the United States
1355100004B/391